AF897045

ESSENTIALS AND CONTROVERSIES IN BARIATRIC SURGERY

Edited by **Chih-Kun Huang**

Essentials and Controversies in Bariatric Surgery
http://dx.doi.org/10.5772/57007
Edited by Chih-Kun Huang

Contributors

Jianchun Yu, Asim Shabbir, Chih-Kun Huang, Peter Crookes, Young Kim, Karen E. Gibbs, Gurdeep S. Matharoo, Erika Renick, John N. Afthinos, Tracey Straker, Maria Rita Marques De Oliveira, Patrícia Fátima Souza Novais, Alex Harley Crisp, Flávia Andreia Marin, Irineu Rasera Junior, Celso Vieira De Souza Leite

Published by InTech

Janeza Trdine 9, 51000 Rijeka, Croatia

Copyright © 2014 InTech

Individual chapters are under their authors' copyright and distributed under the Creative Commons Attribution 3.0 license, which allows users to download, copy and build upon published chapters provided that the authors and publisher are properly credited, which ensures maximum dissemination and a wider impact of the authors' work. Any republication, referencing or personal use of the individual chapters or any of their contents must explicitly identify the original source.

Permission for commercial use of the book as a whole, such as (but not limited to) reprint rights, republication, distribution, sales, translation, and reproduction in any and all forms of media, must always be obtained from InTech.

Notice

Statements and opinions expressed in the chapters are these of the individual contributors and not necessarily those of the editors or publisher. No responsibility is accepted for the accuracy of information contained in the published chapters. The publisher assumes no responsibility for any damage or injury to persons or property arising out of the use of any materials, instructions, methods or ideas contained in the book.

Publishing Process Manager Iva Lipovic

Technical Editor InTech DTP team

Cover InTech Design team

First published October, 2014

Printed in Croatia

Additional hard copies can be obtained from orders@intechopen.com

Essentials and Controversies in Bariatric Surgery, Edited by Chih-Kun Huang

p. cm.

ISBN 978-953-51-1726-1

We are IntechOpen, the world's leading publisher of Open Access books

Built by scientists, for scientists

4,200+
Open access books available

116,000+
International authors and editors

125M+
Downloads

151
Countries delivered to

Our authors are among the
Top 1%
most cited scientists

12.2%
Contributors from top 500 universities

CLARIVATE ANALYTICS
BOOK CITATION INDEX
INDEXED

WEB OF SCIENCE™

Selection of our books indexed in the Book Citation Index
in Web of Science™ Core Collection (BKCI)

Interested in publishing with us?
Contact book.department@intechopen.com

Numbers displayed above are based on latest data collected.
For more information visit www.intechopen.com

For EU product safety concerns :
IN TECH d.o.o., Prolaz Marije Krucifikse Kozulić 3, 51000 Rijeka, Croatia,
info@intechopen.com or visit our website at intechopen.com.

Meet the editor

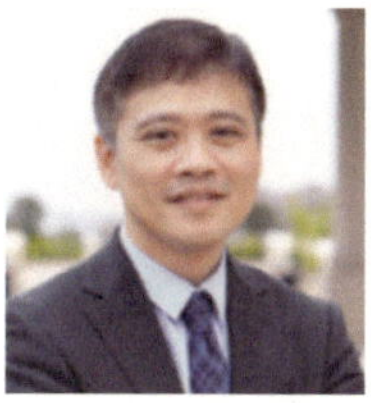

Dr. Chih-Kun Huang is the Founding Chairman of International Excellence Federation (I.E.F) for Bariatric & Metabolic Surgery and President of Taiwan Obesity Support Association (T.O.S.A). He is also the Director of Bariatric & Metabolic International (B.M.I) Surgery Center and Minimally Invasive Surgery Training Center of E-Da hospital, Taiwan. Dr. Huang has been devoted to minimally invasive surgery and bariatric surgery for more than 10 years. He performed and published the 1st single incision trans-umbilical laparoscopic Roux-en-Y gastric bypass in 2008; laparoscopic adjustable gastric banded plication in 2009 and laparoscopic loop duodenaojejunal bypass with sleeve gastrectomy in 2010. His center was also designated as the 1st International Center of Excellence for Bariatric Surgery (I.C.E) in Asia-Pacific area in 2009.

Contents

Preface

Obesity and diabetes have become "Health Bomb", which attack every city in the world, and no country or area are put at exception. Bariatric surgery has been proved to be clinically effective and economically viable for obese people when compared to non-surgical interventions. Advancement of minimally invasive surgery in the last 20 years has made the safety and reliability widely accepted by the public and government systems. Bariatric surgery not only proves its efficacy in marked long-term weight loss, but also aids in achieving substantial improvement or remission of co-morbidities, attributed to metabolic derangement, including type 2 diabetes mellitus (T2DM), hypertension, hyperlipidemia, and obstructive sleep apnea. It also has been proved to reduce long-term mortality and cancer occurrence in morbidly obese patients. Nowadays it is progressing towards the so-called "metabolic surgery," which performs similar surgery in lower body weight to benefit patients with metabolic derangement, particularly T2DM and also teenagers, although some controversies still exist. In this book, we review the fundamental knowledge of bariatric surgery, including preoperative nutrition, selection, and surgical complication. In the second part, new emerging and novel procedures are thoroughly described and discussed. Unquestionably, this book will offer you essentials as well as the latest concepts of bariatric and metabolic surgery.

Chih-Kun Huang
Bariatric & Metabolic International (B.M.I) Surgery Center,
E-Da Hospital, Taiwan

Section 1

Preparation for Bariatric Patients

Chapter 1

Preoperative Evaluation of Bariatric Surgery Patients

Gurdeep S. Matharoo, Erika Renick,
John N. Afthinos, Tracey Straker and
Karen E. Gibbs

Additional information is available at the end of the chapter

http://dx.doi.org/10.5772/58605

1. Introduction

Bariatric surgery has undergone a revolution since its inception in the 1960's. Great strides have been made in technique, safety and outcomes within the past decade and in the face of the advent of newer procedures. This speaks to a better organization of bariatric surgery as a specialty, improved training and the unwavering demand and pursuit of excellence. Despite substantial improvement within the specialty there are a number of comorbid conditions and preoperative findings revealed that necessitate optimization to obtain the best surgical outcomes.

The ultimate goal of bariatric surgery should be to achieve, in as safe a manner as possible, weight loss for the reduction in comorbid conditions and overall long-term effect on mortality and quality of life. A significant contribution to this task has been a more thorough understanding of obesity-related comorbidities and their effects on patient outcomes with respect to perioperative morbidity and mortality. The evaluation of different comorbid conditions through large patient databases has elucidated which comorbid factors contribute towards perioperative morbidity and mortality.

The goal of this chapter will be to review the preoperative evaluation of patients preparing for weight loss surgery. An overview of the general concepts will be described, and then a detailed discussion of the more common comorbid conditions will be presented, along with relevant points and recent literature to support the recommendations. We will utilize an organ system approach. The strategy and rationale for the evaluations that are recommended (or not) will be discussed. Their impact on outcomes will be elucidated for the reader to understand and use to appropriately assess the patient preparing for surgery. An evidence-based approach will show us how to maximize our evaluations of these patients. Awareness of these details

INTECH
open science | open minds

© 2014 The Author(s). Licensee InTech. This chapter is distributed under the terms of the Creative Commons Attribution License (http://creativecommons.org/licenses/by/3.0), which permits unrestricted use, distribution, and reproduction in any medium, provided the original work is properly cited.

empowers healthcare providers to choose and counsel patients appropriately in the preoperative setting.

Weight loss surgery has been shown to have a significant impact on the lives of our patients. Yet, we still face the issue of effectively evaluating and optimizing these patients in the preoperative setting to allow them to partake of the benefits that await them on the other side. The following preoperative evaluations will be addressed in the chapter: indications, cardiovascular, vascular (venous system), pulmonary, endocrine, gastrointestinal, nutritional, psychological, education, functional status. The significance of the final evaluation by the anesthesiologist will also be discussed. Irrespective of the procedure chosen (gastric bypass, gastric bypass, sleeve gastrectomy, duodenal switch), approach used (laparoscopic or open) the preoperative evaluation is essential to prepare the patient for this major lifestyle change.

2. Indications

In 1991 the National Institutes of Health published a consensus statement regarding weight loss surgery. Surgery was indicated in patients with a BMI ≥ 40 kg/m^2 and in patients with a BMI between 35 and 40 if they also had comorbidities. Severe sleep apnea, Pickwickian syndrome, obesity related cardiomyopathy, severe diabetes mellitus and lifestyle limitations were all considered comorbidities that would allow the patient to pursue surgery [1]. Since 1991 significant strides have been made in the field of weight loss surgery. It has since been proven to be a method for sustained weight loss and resolution of comorbid conditions. As the benefits to surgery continually develop, movements to change the indications to allow for more patients to achieve the benefits of weight loss have been published. In 2009, recommendations were made to expand the indications to both adolescent (12 – 18 years old) and elderly (>65 years old) patients [2].

For patients with a BMI ≥ 40 kg/m^2, surgery is indicated for ages 19 – 64, even without comorbid conditions. Adolescents with a BMI ≥ 40 kg/m^2 must have prediabetes, diabetes with Hgb A_{1c} > 9, regardless of therapy or 7-9 on maximal medical therapy, severe hypertension (SBP > 140 and DBP > 90), hyperlipidemia, any degree of sleep apnea or joint pain interfering with daily life in order to qualify for surgery. Elderly patients with BMI ≥ 40, like adolescents, require comorbid conditions to qualify for surgery. The presence of diabetes with Hgb A_{1c} > 9, regardless of therapy or 7-9 on maximal medical therapy, hypertension, hyperlipidemia, moderate to severe sleep apnea, venous stasis, or severe chronic joint pain would indicate the need for weight loss surgery.

Patients with a BMI 35 – 39 kg/m^2 and aged 19 – 64 should be recommended for surgery as outlined in the 1991 NIH consensus statement. For adolescents in this BMI range diabetes with Hgb A_{1c} > 7, refractory severe hypertension or moderate to severe sleep apnea are required to proceed with surgery. In the elderly population with BMI 35 – 39 kg/m^2, diabetes with Hgb A_{1c} > 9, regardless of therapy or 7-9 on maximal medical therapy, refractory hypertension, and moderate to severe sleep apnea are all criterion which support proceeding to surgery.

Around the world, the indications for surgery differ based on the populations and prevalence of obesity related comorbidities. In Europe, the guidelines allow for surgery in patients with a BMI ≥40 kg/m^2, BMI ≥ 35 kg/m^2 with severe comorbidities, BMI 30-35 kg/m^2 with diabetes, in adolescents if BMI ≥ 40 kg/m^2 and in the elderly with a favorable risk to benefit profile [3]. In the Asian population, the visceral fat percentage is higher than in Caucasian persons [4]. Asian persons also have a higher risk of developing diabetes mellitus, hypertension and hyperlipidemia at a lower BMI relative to persons of other ethnicities. These factors support the guidelines in Asia where surgery is recommended for all patients with a BMI ≥ 35 kg/m^2. Surgery is also considered for patients with a BMI > 30 kg/m^2 with diabetes mellitus or metabolic syndrome and inability to control with lifestyle alterations or medications [5].

3. Cardiovascular

Obesity has a negative effect on cardiovascular health. The presence of obesity increases the risk for coronary artery disease, heart failure, cardiomyopathy, atrial fibrillation and hypertension [6]. All of these conditions, if not optimized, can lead to poor surgical outcomes in bariatric surgery patients.

The approach to perioperative cardiovascular evaluation for non-cardiac surgery has been extensively studied. The general principle to follow is that intervention is rarely needed in order to lower risk unless it is indicated irrespective of the perioperative context [7]. There are clinical predictors which place patients into categories based on risk of perioperative cardiac events. Major predictors are unstable coronary syndromes, acute or recent myocardial infarction with ongoing ischemic risk factors, unstable or severe angina, decompensated heart failure, significant arrhythmias, high-grade atrio-ventricular blocks, certain arrhythmias and severe valvular disease. Intermediate predictors include mild angina pectoris, previous myocardial infarctions, compensated or prior heart failure, diabetes mellitus and renal insufficiency. Minor predictors are advanced age, abnormal ECG, rhythm other than sinus, low functional capacity, uncontrolled systemic hypertension and previous stroke. The type of surgery is also associated with cardiac risk. Bariatric surgery is considered an intermediate risk procedure.

Hypertension is found in 13.8 to 25.7 percent of obese patients [8,9]. In patients with stage three hypertension, systolic blood pressure ≥180 mm Hg and a diastolic blood pressure ≥ 110 mm Hg, the risk of proceeding with surgery must be evaluated [7]. Presence of hypertension as a comorbidity is an independent risk factor for mortality after open or laparoscopic gastric bypass with an odds ratio of 2.783 [10]. Treatment with beta blockers has been shown to decrease the risk of myocardial infarction and cardiovascular death in high risk patients [11]. When indicated, beta blockers should be initiated several weeks prior to surgery and titrated to achieve a resting heart rate of 50 to 60 beats per minute [12]. As bariatric surgery is an elective procedure, we recommend delaying surgery until adequate blood pressure control is achieved. Hypertension should be controlled before surgery with continuation of the preoperative antihypertensive treatment through the perioperative period [7]. Caution is advised when preparing a patient taking clonidine or beta blockers for surgery, due to known rebound hypertension upon abrupt discontinuation. These antihypertensive agents may be converted to transdermal or intravenous forms, respectively, during the time a patient is nil per os (NPO)[11]. Continuation of beta blockers through the perioperative period is recommended in those patients being treated for angina, specific arrhythmias, hypertension and other American College of Cardiology (ACC)/ American Heart Association (AHA) Class 1 guideline indications [7].

The myriad of available tests to assess cardiac function can be overwhelming and choosing which test to order can be confusing. Generally evaluation begins with a 12-lead electrocardiogram (ECG). In bariatric surgery patients ECG abnormalities can uncover predictors of perioperative and long term cardiovascular risk. ECG is recommended in all patients who have had a recent episode of chest pain, asymptomatic patients with diabetes mellitus, patients with prior coronary revascularization, asymptomatic males over 45 years old or females over 55 years old with two or more atherosclerotic risk factors and those patients who have had prior hospital admissions for cardiac causes [7]. Further evaluation of cardiac function involves stress testing and coronary angiography. Both methods are geared towards identifying patients with cardiac ischemia.

Exercise or pharmacological stress testing is recommended in adult patients with intermediate pretest probability of coronary artery disease based on ECG, those undergoing initial evaluation for suspected or proven coronary artery disease and patients with a significant change in clinical status. Exercise testing is also useful to evaluate exercise capacity when subjective measures are unreliable [7]. Some patients will not tolerate an exercise stress test. In this group of patients a pharmacological stress test should be considered. Noninvasive cardiac imaging without the use of pharmacological stressing agents is able to provide visualization of left ventricular function at rest. Although this test is commonly done during preoperative evaluations it is not a consistent predictor of perioperative ischemic events. Non-invasive stress testing, such as a dobutamine stress echocardiogram, is able to predict perioperative cardiac events by visualizing the amount of myocardium at risk for ischemia [7]. It has been shown, however, that the accuracy of thallium-201 nuclear cardiac imaging can be diminished in patients who have a BMI over 30 kg/m^2, which is specific to our patient population [13]. There is mounting evidence that cardiac computed tomography angiogram can be used as a method to evaluate the coronary vasculature in patients unable to tolerate exercise prior to invasive imaging procedures [14].

Coronary angiography is the definitive test for intraluminal causes of cardiac ischemia. The procedure is diagnostic and can also be therapeutic with the usage of balloon angioplasty with or without stent placement. Coronary angioplasty should be done on patients with suspected or known coronary artery disease. These patients have a high risk of adverse outcome based on noninvasive test results, angina unresponsive to adequate medical therapy or unstable angina [7]. Percutaneous coronary intervention (PCI) does not decrease the risk of perioperative cardiac events except in those patients in whom PCI is indicated for acute coronary syndrome. Although the PCI can reduce perioperative cardiac events, one of the major limitations of treatment is the subsequent delay in surgery due to the direct mechanical effects of angioplasty or the required anti platelet therapy. Patients who undergo PCI with balloon therapy alone should undergo surgery between four and eight weeks after catheterization. Before four weeks the dilated blood vessels have not fully healed and after eight weeks the risk of restenosis is high [7].

Cardiac medications after coronary artery stenting present a controversy for the surgeon as the drugs increase the risk of bleeding during the perioperative period. Stent placement requires dual anti platelet therapy with clopidogrel and aspirin in the post PCI period to prevent stent thrombosis. The American College of Cardiology and The American Heart Association recommend that dual anti platelet treatment is required for at least one month in patients receiving bare metal stents and for one year with drug eluting stents [7]. In a literature review currently in press, the authors examined the perioperative management of anti platelet therapy and they found variability among the recommendations. However, they recommend delaying surgery for at least four to twelve weeks in patients with bare metal stents. In patients with drug eluting stents they recommend postponing surgery for at least six to twelve months [15]. Specific to elective surgery, such as the bariatric population, Katkhouda et al recommends that patients with bare metal or drug eluting stents should not undergo surgery within the first year of stent placement. If, as determined by a cardiologist, the patient requires dual therapy longer than one year after stent placement, clopidogrel and other thienopyridines should be stopped five to ten days preoperatively and restarted ten days postoperatively [12]. The continuation of aspirin through the perioperative period is recommended [12,15]. In patients undergoing gastric bypass it is recommended to start proton pump inhibitors one week preoperatively and subsequently continue them through the perioperative period to minimize the risk of gastrointestinal bleeding upon restarting clopidogrel therapy [12].

Management of valvular heart disease is dependent on the pathophysiology of the valve. Patients with symptomatic aortic stenosis should have their surgery delayed and undergo valve replacement prior to non-cardiac surgery. If the patient has severe stenosis but is asymptomatic the aortic valve should be evaluated with imaging. Patients unwilling or unable to undergo cardiac surgery for severe aortic stenosis have a 10% mortality rate from non-cardiac surgery. With mild or moderate mitral valve stenosis, the heart rate must be controlled during the perioperative period to minimize pulmonary congestion created by decreased diastolic filling times. Patients with significant mitral stenosis are at risk for heart failure during the perioperative period. Operative correction of mitral stenosis is not recommended unless the valvular condition should be corrected to prolong survival and prevent complications that are unrelated to the non-cardiac surgery [11].

Congestive heart failure (CHF) has been found to be a significant factor in perioperative cardiac events. The preoperative evaluation must include screening for CHF which can be done with history and physical exam alone – look for prior history of heart failure, symptoms of paroxysmal nocturnal dyspnea, presence of an S3 gallop, jugular venous distention, peripheral edema, bilateral rales on lung auscultation and evidence of pulmonary vascular redistribution on chest x-ray [11]. The Framingham Heart Study identified obesity as an independent risk factor for the development of heart failure; with the risk increasing by 5% in men and 7% in women for every 1 kg/m^2 in BMI [16]. The optimal treatment for CHF is determined by identifying the cause and degree of failure.

Close collaboration with the patient's cardiologist during the preoperative workup can allow for a smooth progression through preoperative cardiac testing, while accurately assessing and optimizing risk factors.

4. Venous

Venous thromboembolic events (VTE) continue to be one of the most significant postoperative complications after weight loss surgery; the other being staple line leaks and the associated septic sequelae. Obesity is considered a hypercoagulable state. The odds ratio of VTE is between 1.97 and 2.39 in those with a BMI greater than 30 kg/m^2 [17]. Bariatric surgery has been also been associated with a hypercoagulable state due to increased levels of clotting factors during the perioperative period from surgical trauma [18,19]. VTE events are a leading cause for mortality after bariatric surgery [20]. It is generally recommended that patients undergoing weight loss surgery receive VTE prophylaxis during the perioperative period. Postoperative ambulation and lower extremity sequential compression devices are safe and recommended for all bariatric patients when appropriate. The proper use of chemoprophylaxis and the preoperative insertion of inferior vena cava (IVC) filters have been controversial.

The identification of deep venous thrombosis is fundamental to preventing further complications from clot progression or embolus. The preferred method for evaluation is venous duplex ultrasound. This study has a sensitivity and specificity of 97% and 94%, respectively, of diagnosing a proximal lower extremity DVT [21]. Traditionally, many bariatric centers included this exam as part of the preoperative workup. A five year retrospective review of our own bariatric patient population revealed that only one of 555 patients (0.2%) was found to have a DVT on preoperative workup. This patient had a history of a chronic DVT, known prior to the examination. Our findings coincided with two previous studies which also showed that no preoperative investigation is needed [22,23]. Based on these finding we do not recommend routine preoperative venous duplex ultrasound; however, testing may be warranted in patients with prior history of DVT or significant venous insufficiency.

The preoperative placement of inferior vena cava (IVC) filters has been reported in high risk bariatric surgery patients. In some institutions, it was routine to have an IVC filter placed in patients with BMI greater than 55 kg/m^2, immobility, venous stasis, pulmonary hypertension, obesity hypoventilation syndrome, hypercoagulability, and a history of VTE [20]. It was recommended that patients with BMI greater than 55 kg/m^2 undergoing open gastric bypass undergo placement of IVC filter while those having laparoscopic surgery could forego the filter placement [24,25]. Recently, however, the routine use of IVC filters has undergone scrutiny. The Michigan Bariatric Surgery Collaborative (MBSC) published the largest series to date regarding the efficacy of preoperative IVC filters in gastric bypass patients. They found that there was no difference in the rates of VTE, serious complications and death or permanent disability [26]. In the same month, the United States Food and Drug Administration (FDA) published an advisory report regarding the use of retrievable IVC filters. They highlighted 921 device related adverse events since 2005. The FDA recommended a judicious approach to placement and vigilant follow up for prompt removal of IVC filters [27]. This prompted another study from the MBSC to investigate outcomes in patients treated with IVC filters. They discovered that patients with IVC filters had worse outcomes than comparable patients without IVC filters. A significant number of patients with IVC filters were also subjected to device related complications, such as thrombosis and occlusion, filter migration, contrast induced nephropathy and incision site infection. They found the rate of DVT and VTE were significantly higher in patients with IVC filters, odds ratios 2.7 and 3.3, respectively. Furthermore, there was no difference in the rates of pulmonary embolus between the groups. They concluded that IVC filters do not reduce the risk of pulmonary embolism in high risk bariatric surgery patients and that their use should be discouraged in bariatric surgery patients [28].

Chemoprophylaxis is generally achieved with subcutaneous injections of unfractionated heparin (UFH) or low molecular weight heparin (LMWH). Since patients are most susceptible to venous stasis during the induction of anesthesia, the first dose of chemoprophylaxis should be given preoperatively [29]. Our patients receive 5,000 units of unfractionated heparin administered subcutaneously immediately prior to entering the operating room. All patients are also treated with bilateral lower extremity sequential compression devices, which are placed prior to induction of anesthesia. This combination of chemical and mechanical prophylaxis has been shown to limit the development of deep venous thrombosis and bleeding complications [22]. Dosages and frequency vary among the different formulations of low molecular weight heparinoids, as does their method of action. A recent literature review concluded that there are three "standard regimens" for chemoprophylaxis of VTE – UFH 5000 units 2 – 3 daily, LMWH 30 mg twice daily, 40 mg once daily or weight adjusted LMWH [30]. The authors concluded that there was no difference in the rate of VTE among the different regimens, but the use of weight adjusted dosing increased the risk of major bleeding.

Patients with a history of heparin induced thrombocytopenia (HIT) type 2 present a unique challenge in VTE prophylaxis. This population has not been studied in bariatric surgery; however, VTE prophylaxis in the orthopedic population with HIT type 2 is accomplished by the use of desirudin administered subcutaneously [31]. More investigation is needed to recommend this medication usage beyond the specialty of orthopedics.

5. Pulmonary

Obesity related impairment of respiratory function is caused by mechanical restriction of adequate ventilation. The increased adipose tissue reduces diaphragmatic excursion, chest wall expansion and oropharyngeal patency. Obesity is also a risk factor for airway disease and there is a 50% higher incidence of severe asthma in obese patients when compared to normal controls [32,33].

A reduction in the expiratory reserve volume (ERV) is the most commonly identified abnormality on spirometry. Both body mass index and body fat distribution contribute to the degree of decrease in ERV. Hamoui et al has shown that in patients undergoing open duodenal switch procedures there is a relative risk of 2.29 to develop postoperative complications for every 10% decrease in percent of predicted value of vital capacity (VC). They also found that patients with a VC of less than 80% of predicted have a 54.5% prevalence of postoperative complications [34].

The increased rate of complications was also found in laparoscopic bariatric surgery. In 2013, van Huisstede et al prospectively examined their patients undergoing laparoscopic gastric bypass and laparoscopic sleeve gastrectomy. Among the 485 patients studied, they found patients with airflow obstruction ($FEV_1/FVC < 70\%$) or airflow reversibility (change in $FEV_1 > 12\%$) after administration of a bronchodilator, had an increased risk of postoperative complications with an adjusted odds ratio of 2.9 [35]. They recommend spirometry be done routinely on all patients being evaluated for bariatric surgery. The authors of this chapter follow these recommendations and routinely evaluate all patients with preoperative pulmonary function tests.

As pulmonary function tests are often abnormal in obese patients, the causes for abnormality must be identified and optimized prior to surgery [34]. Smoking is a common entity which significantly impacts pulmonary function therefore smoking cessation is an essential component of the preoperative assessment. In a study of over 300,000 patients from the Nationwide Inpatient Sample database smoking was identified as an independent factor associated with a greater incidence of acute respiratory failure after bariatric surgery [36]. Smoking has also been shown to be an independent predictor of increased hospital length of stay. Current and past smokers have been shown to require four and one days longer in the hospital, respectively, than patients that never smoked [37]. Nicotine, in all forms, is known to have vasoconstrictor properties. This may add to the microvascular disease caused by smoking which has been reported to increase the incidence of marginal ulceration and gastrointestinal anastomotic dehiscence [38,39]. It is our recommendation to not offer surgery to patients who are current smokers and to those using a nicotine replacement in an attempt to quit smoking. It is our practice to require smoking cessation to minimize the above mentioned morbidities.

Obstructive sleep apnea (OSA) is a condition in which the upper airway periodically becomes narrowed or obstructed during sleep and results in reduction or cessation of breathing during sleep. The reduction in airway caliber is due to the sleep induced loss of muscle tone in the soft tissues of the oropharyngeal airway. Obstructive sleep apnea is found in 38 – 88% of morbidly obese patients [40]. There are many screening tools available to the bariatric surgeon to identify patients at risk for having OSA. The Epworth Sleepiness Score, the Maintenance of Wakefulness Test, the Berlin Questionnaire and the STOP-BANG Questionnaire are designed to quickly asses if a patient should be screened further. The definitive diagnosis of OSA is made with an overnight polysomnography. The test measures the number of hypopnea (30% or greater decrease in airflow for at least 10 seconds followed by an arousal and/or 3% oxygen desaturation) and apnea (complete or near complete cessation of airflow for at least 10 seconds followed by an arousal and/or 3% oxygen desaturation) events and results with an 'apnea hypopnea index', which is classified to the severity of the sleep apnea [41]. Nonoperative treatment of OSA is achieved with non invasive positive pressure ventilation in the form of continuous positive airway pressure (CPAP) or bi-level positive airway pressure (Bi-PAP). Many patients receive the diagnosis for the first time during the preoperative work up for bariatric surgery. These patients should be allowed to adapt to the device prior to undergoing surgery. With regards to anastomotic integrity, the use of CPAP has been proven to be safe after roux-en-y gastric bypass [42]. In order to maximize compliance, patients should bring their own machine and mask to the hospital. Although the use of CPAP or BiPAP is recommended in the postoperative setting, its omission has also been proven safe provided the patient is an a monitored setting with aggressive pulmonary physiotherapy [40].

In addition to OSA, patients with super morbid obesity can have pulmonary derangements while awake; this is termed obesity hypoventilation syndrome (OHS). More specifically, obesity hypoventilation syndrome manifests with daytime hypercapnia with $PaCO_2 > 44$ mm Hg or 6 kPa, elevated hematocrit, and sleep disordered breathing. These patients are at high risk for pulmonary complications and VTE [40]. Obesity hypoventilation syndrome occurs in 11% of patients with OSA and in 8% of bariatric surgical patients [43]. Patients with OHS have severe upper airway obstruction, impaired respiratory mechanics, blunted central respiratory drive and increased incidence of pulmonary hypertension. The diagnosis of OHS is also made with polysomnography. The treatment of OHS is similar to OSA in that positive airway pressure and supplemental oxygen are used to facilitate adequate respiration.

We reviewed our patient database and found that approximately 85% of patients had undiagnosed obstructive sleep apnea with 51% of patients having severe sleep apnea. In the lower BMI range (35-39.9 kg/m^2) our population showed 92% prevalence of OSA. There was a 100% prevalence of obstructive sleep apnea in those with a BMI greater than or equal to 60 kg/m^2. Based on these results, we can see that BMI does not correlate with the presence of OSA. In a larger study of 2,458 patients, 509 patients underwent polysomnography within one year prior to bariatric surgery. In this population 80.7% of patients were found to have obstructive sleep apnea and 35.5% of these patients had severe sleep apnea [44]. Although some authors advise that polysomnography should only be used if the patient exhibits symptoms of OSA or OHS, we recommend that all patients be actively evaluated with polysomnography in the preoperative period. If found to have sleep apnea, the patients are started on positive pressure ventilation by mask, at the settings recommended, for several weeks prior to surgery. On the day of the surgery, the patient is instructed to bring their machine to the hospital and the machine is routinely used, starting in the recovery room.

6. Anesthesia

The anesthesia preoperative assessment is the culmination of all consults pertinent to the optimization of the physiological status of the patient. Provided that major cardiopulmonary issues, cerebral, and metabolic derangements have been addressed, the anesthesiologist should be able to proceed with the surgery in a controlled and safe manner. As the preoperative optimization of these organ systems have been addressed previously in this chapter, the focus of the anesthesiology section will be intravenous access, blood pressure monitoring, aspiration risk, and airway management on induction of anesthesia.

Peripheral intravenous access in the bariatric patient may be difficult. The anesthesiologist should be prepared to use ultrasound guided techniques or central venous access placement in patients where intravenous access is difficult. Arterial line placement may be utilized when an appropriately sized blood pressure cuff may not reflect accurate readings secondary to the conical shaped arms in this population [45]. The possibility of central line placement preoperatively should be discussed with the patient prior to going into the operating room.

Airway management during anesthesia induction may be challenging in the bariatric population. BMI ≥ to 40 kg/m^2 has been associated with significant airway management challenges. Some institutions have mandated having an attending and one other experienced anesthesia provider (attending, an anesthesia resident with floor intubation credentialing, or CRNA available for intubation in this population). Due to excess soft tissue related to the anatomy, face mask ventilation of the morbidly obese patient may be difficult. Increased BMI and a history of OSA also increase the possibility of difficult face mask ventilation [46]. When a Mallampati 3 or 4 score is assessed, there has been increased difficulty in intubation, see figure 1 [47].

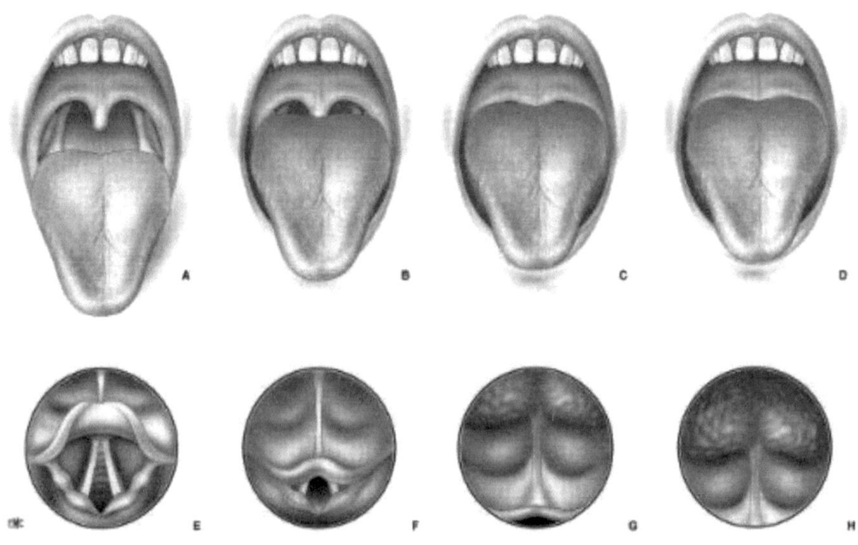

Figure 1. Mallampati Classification and Laryngoscopic View Grades.

Positioning of the bariatric patient in the supine position, as seen in figure 2, such that the external auditory meatus is in line with the sternal notch, known as ramping, is recommended [48]. A recent study demonstrated that in the morbidly obese population undergoing bariatric surgery, when using the "ramping" position, there was no correlation between difficult direct laryngoscopy and OSA in Mallampati 1 and 2 classifications. Patients with a BMI of 35kg/m2 have been associated with a greater than 6 fold increase in difficult direct laryngoscopy. Neck circumference over 40 cm has also been implicated in difficult direct laryngoscopy [49].

http://dx.doi.org/10.5772/58605

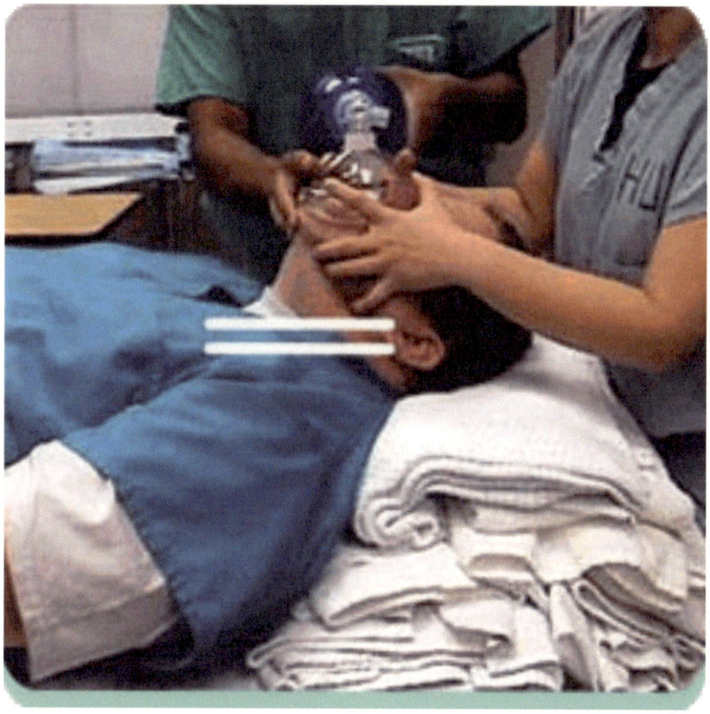

Figure 2. Ramping position.

In addition to ventilation and intubation concerns, aspiration risk must be considered. It has been reported that the gastric fluid of morbidly obese patients is more voluminous and of lower pH than that of the leaner patients [50]. These patients can be considered for rapid sequence induction, a technique for inducing a patient without ventilation. This technique may expose the anesthesiologist to a greater chance of airway failure. Neutralization of gastric acid with clear antacid solutions such as sodium citrate can be prophylactically given preoperatively.

There are many adjunct airway devices available to assist in the intubation of a challenging airway. The advent of video laryngoscopy, a plethora of supraglottic airways and flexible fiber optic intubation has provided multiple modalities and techniques for intubation of the challenging airway.

When assessing the airway of the bariatric patient, a preoperative plan for securing the airway safely is invaluable. The American Society of Anesthesiology (ASA) Difficult Airway Algorithm gives several pathways for the management of the difficult airway, whether the patient is awake or asleep, see figure 3 [51].

If the anesthesiologist's evaluation raises doubt in the ability to safely manage the airway, awake intubation should be undertaken [52]. It is also important to remember that BMI alone does not predict the probability of a difficult intubation. Preparedness, vigilance and communication with the surgeon will result in a favorable patient outcome.

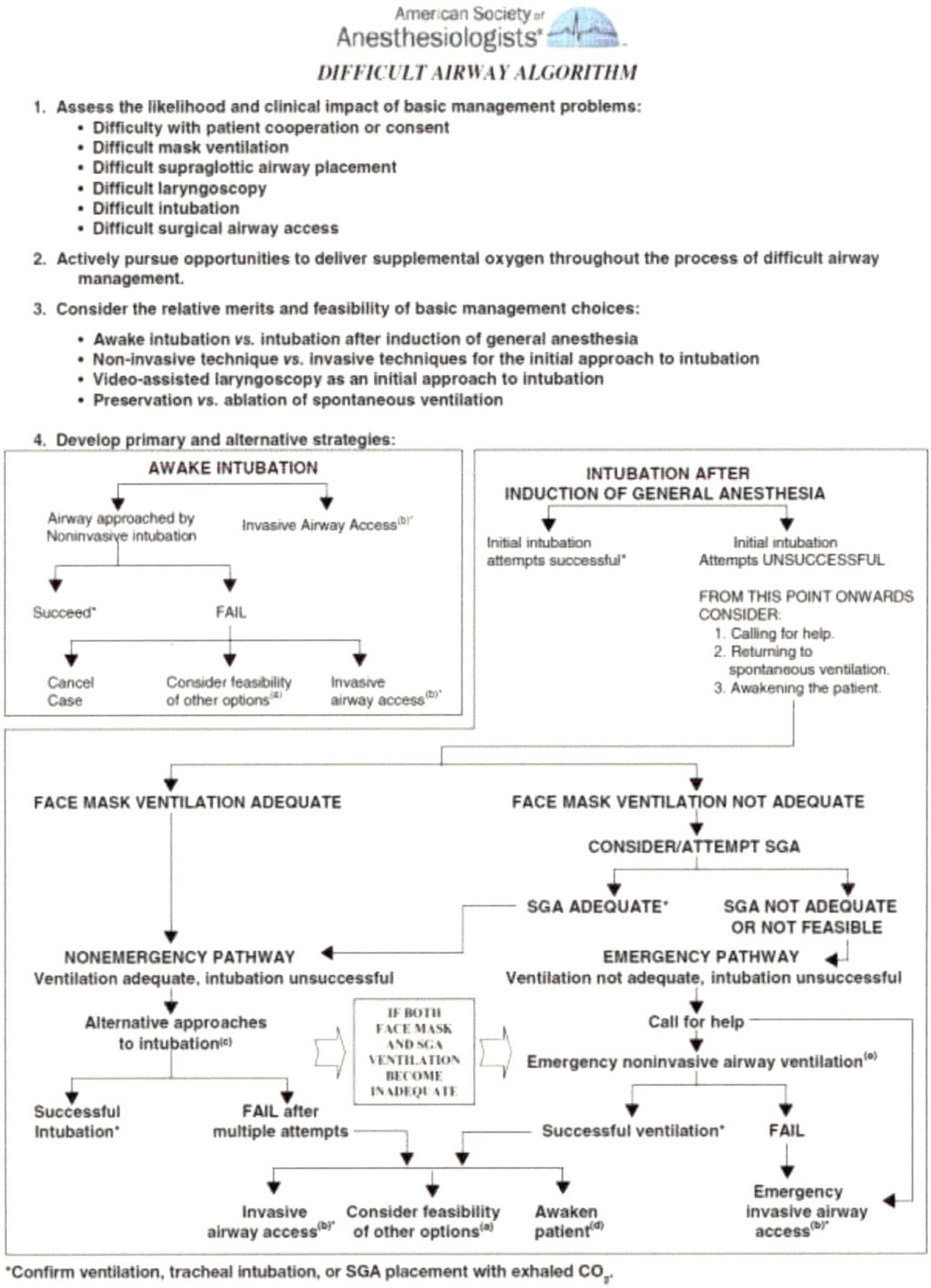

Figure 3. Difficult Airway Algorithm.

7. Endocrine

Evidence is accumulating that suggests obesity is closely related to endocrine disorders, some at a subclinical level. Obesity has been found to be associated with type 2 diabetes mellitus (T2DM) and hypothyroidism [53,54].

Management of T2DM is important during the perioperative period. Targets have been established by the American Association of Clinical Endocrinologists, The Obesity Society and the American Society for Metabolic and Bariatric Surgery for preoperative glycemic control which may be associated with improved outcomes, see table 1 [53].

• Hemoglobin A_{1c} of 6.5 – 7.0 % or less
• Fasting blood glucose level of less than or equal to 110 mg/dL
•2-hour postprandial blood glucose concentration of less than or equal to 140 ml/dL

Table 1. Recommendations for preoperative glycemic control

Optimal glycemic control should be achieved preoperatively, as patients with an elevated preoperative hemoglobin A_{1c} are found to have a higher incidence of postoperative complications. A hemoglobin A_{1c} level greater than 8% increases the risk of wound infection and acute renal failure postoperatively. An elevated A_{1c} in the preoperative setting also increases the likelihood of elevated blood glucose in the postoperative setting and decreases the rate of resolution of T2DM after bariatric surgery [55]. Preoperative control can be achieved with a combination of diet modification, weight loss and pharmaceuticals.

Hypothyroidism is a known cause of obesity; however, de novo thyroid dysfunction has been observed in obese patients. It has been suggested that subclinical hypothyroidism is associated with obesity [54]. In some patients, the TSH level has been shown to return to normal levels after significant weight loss, however the outcome is not universal. The ASMBS does not recommend routine screening for primary hypothyroidism in the obese patients, however many bariatric programs require such preoperative screening in keeping with the NIH guidelines to ensure there is no organic cause to the obesity [53,56].

8. Gastrointestinal

Obesity is a risk factor for gastroesophageal reflux disease, erosive esophagitis, and esophageal adenocarcinoma [57]. The presence of gastrointestinal diseases has an effect on the type of bariatric procedure, which can be recommended for a patient and may require treatment prior to weight loss surgery. In addition, after surgery, the restrictions and rearrangement of the alimentary tract can limit evaluation and surveillance options. There are many modalities for assessing the gastrointestinal tract in the preoperative setting.

The American Society for Gastrointestinal Endoscopy (ASGE) recommends an upper endoscopy be performed in all patients with upper GI tract symptoms and in all patients undergoing weight loss surgery [58]. Preoperative esophagogastroduodenoscopy has been found to reveal abnormalities in 46 to 90% of patients, with 62% having clinically significant findings. In our practice, all patients being evaluated for bariatric surgery undergo upper endoscopy. However, a five year, internal review of 555 patients has shown 98% of our patients had positive findings on routine upper endoscopy yet the findings did not cause a delay or impact on the choice of surgical procedure – questioning the clinical significance of the findings.

During endoscopy tissue biopsies should be obtained to evaluate for *H. pylori.* If the bacterium is isolated, eradication with one of several standard regimens is recommended. Recently, there has been growing support for non-invasive testing for *H. pylori* in an effort to reduce costs associated with preoperative testing [59]. One potential algorithm for non-invasive testing involves screening patients with serum *H. pylori* test and treating the patient if it is positive. In either case, proof of eradication should be obtained, typically via urea breath test. Recently published data indicates that preoperative *H. pylori* status does not increase the risk for marginal ulcer or stomal stenosis post roux-en-y gastric bypass [60].

The World Health Organization (WHO) reports the incidence of gastric cancer is highest in the western pacific region, which comprises 27 countries including China, Japan, Republic of Korea, Malaysia, Singapore and the Philippines. The incidence in this region was 521,000 cases in 2004, greater than 50% of the worldwide incidence [61]. In countries where gastric and other upper gastrointestinal cancers are more prevalent, the importance of preoperative upper endoscopy cannot be underestimated. Ultimately, practice patterns should reflect the prevalence of significant findings specific to the patient population being prepared for weight loss surgery.

As an adjunct to endoscopic examination of the gastrointestinal tract several radiographic investigations are also considered during the preoperative evaluation for bariatric surgery. Gastroesophageal reflux disease associated with hiatal hernias is commonly found in obese patients. Completing a bariatric procedure without recognizing and repairing a hiatal hernia can potentially lead to worsening of reflux and poor surgical outcomes [62]. In order to identify a hiatal hernia some surgeons obtain contrast enhanced upper GI series. We do not employ upper GI series routinely in our preoperative evaluations. Hiatal hernias that are identified on preoperative upper endoscopy are discussed with the patient for informed consent and subsequently investigated during the operation. In our experience, clinically significant hiatal hernias are readily identifiable upon laparoscopic inspection and repaired as indicated.

In our practice we routinely assess the size of the liver prior to surgery by abdominal ultrasound. Greater than 30% of morbidly obese patient show fatty infiltration of the liver [63]. As an enlarged liver is one of the most common reasons for conversion to an open procedure, it is our practice to place the patient on a liquid diet for two weeks prior to surgery if hepatic steatosis is identified [64]. Two weeks of a low energy diet has been shown to decrease liver size and body fat by greater than 5% [63]. In addition to liver size, the gallbladder is also evaluated for the presence of stones and wall thickening to suggest chronic gallstone disease. The management of concurrent gallstones in the morbidly obese patient undergoing bariatric surgery has been a controversial topic. During the era of open weight loss surgery concomitant cholecystectomy was recommended for all patients undergoing open gastric bypass [65,66].

The view on cholecystectomy has changed since the widespread adoption of laparoscopic bariatric surgery. Addition of cholecystectomy to laparoscopic roux-en-y gastric bypass was found to add approximately 50 minutes to the operative time and significantly increased hospital length of stay, 2.69 days versus 4.35 days [67]. A study of 625 patients by D'Hount et al showed that only 6.9% of patients developed symptomatic gallstone disease post gastric bypass. The mean time between gastric bypass and cholecystectomy was 17.4 ± 13.1 months [68]. We do not advocate performing cholecystectomy at the same time as primary bariatric procedures unless absolutely necessary due to the increased operative time and length of stay. We do employ the use of ursodeoxycholic acid in the postoperative period to reduce the rate of gallstone formation in our gastric bypass patients due to the challenge of addressing choledocholithiasis in this patient population [53].

9. Nutritional

A preoperative nutritional assessment with a registered dietitian is essential when preparing for surgery. The preoperative nutritional assessment is designed to help the patient recognize the need for positive lifestyle changes and develop a plan to implement them. This will likely result in improvement of nutritional status, better management of nutrition-related comorbidities and development of habits that will positively influence weight loss outcomes and maintenance [69]. It is also a time to thoroughly review the postoperative diet with the patient, which includes gradually advancing the diet in terms of texture and variety, including exercise on a regular basis, staying hydrated with appropriate fluids, and adhering to the recommended vitamin and mineral regimen. In this section, we will discuss preoperative behavior changes that could potentially affect long-term outcomes.

A thorough preoperative nutritional assessment should include review of anthropometrical data, weight history, past diet history, medical history, available laboratory values, psychological history (including history of eating disorders), social history, substance abuse history, nutrition-focused physical findings (such as poor dentition), dietary intake, physical activity, and psychosocial factors that affect weight loss [70]. When discussing dietary intake with a patient, it is important to determine how many meals the patient includes on a daily basis, whether or not the patient snacks all day (i.e. grazing, picking, nibbling), if the patient has a past or current history of eating disorders, macronutrient and micronutrient composition of frequently chosen foods and beverages, and alcohol intake [69]. Preoperative nutrition counseling should be adapted to each individual patient.

Patients' eating habits and exercise patterns are determined by a variety of environmental, psychological, biological, and social factors. Environmental factors include work schedule, occupation, socioeconomic status, and family traditions. Psychological factors include low self-esteem, feeling a lack of control in life, feeling inadequate, depression, anxiety, stress, and loneliness. Social factors include cultural glorification of the "perfect body", society placing more value on physical appearance and not on inner qualities, and stress related to size/body shape due to past discrimination [71]. Biological and biochemical factors are still being explored, but recent research has shown that gastrointestinal hormone imbalance can affect hunger and appetite [72]. It is important for patients to understand that, regardless of the reasons behind them, current eating patterns will likely result in poor weight loss, weight regain, and malnutrition after surgery. Preoperative nutritional counseling should focus on addressing these behaviors, working with the patient to avoid or manage them, and having the patient demonstrate compliance with the recommended changes.

Two environmental factors that are of particular concern are socioeconomic status and shift work. In low-income areas, access to nutrient-rich foods is oftentimes limited [73]. Planning grocery lists and affordable recipes with a low-income patient would be an appropriate intervention. Having the patient complete food logs that show more meals are prepared in the home with the ingredients purchased from the grocery list will demonstrate that he/she is able to incorporate this healthy behavior on a routine basis, thus lowering the risk of postoperative malnutrition. Obesity is frequently seen in people who work overnight shifts or who have alternating shifts and late shift workers have higher rates of weight gain after starting their jobs [74,75]. In our practice, patients report that they feel it is inappropriate to eat in the middle of the night. This often results in eating large portions before work and after work, as well as grazing on empty-calorie foods during the night. Working with the patient to break the idea that it is "bad" to be eating in the night is key when it comes to changing behaviors to positively affect weight loss and nutrition status postoperatively. Including regularly-timed meals and snacks that include an appropriate balance of protein, carbohydrates, and fat will set the patient up for long-term success.

Sometimes, patients have a past or present history of eating disorders that likely require additional psychological counseling in addition to nutritional counseling. Hence, coordination between the dietitian and the mental health care provider is critical. There is a fair amount of literature regarding Binge Eating Disorder (BED), subdiagnostic BED, and night eating syndrome in the preoperative setting, most of which states that psychological counseling is encouraged for patients that have either been diagnosed with an eating disorder or show tendencies towards one [76-78]. Some studies have suggested that patients with preoperative BED might be more inclined to graze after surgery, thus sabotaging weight loss, while other research suggests that prior history of eating disorders is not a predictor of poor outcomes following bariatric surgery [78,79]. Emotional eating is technically not considered an eating disorder, but its presence oftentimes has psychological roots. Some case studies have shown that cognitive behavioral therapy can help manage emotional eating both pre and postoperatively [80]. The only eating disorder that is a contraindication to bariatric surgery is active bulimia nervosa, but ultimately it is up to the multidisciplinary bariatric surgery team to decide if they feel a patient's past history of eating disorders could potentially jeopardize the patient's health [78]. Bariatric surgical teams should keep in mind that the psychological evaluation is not the only setting in which a patient might disclose episodes of disordered eating. Questions inquiring about eating disorders should be included in the nutrition evaluation, and if during subsequent visits the patient suggests that he or she has tendencies towards these behaviors, the patient should undergo psychological treatment before proceeding with surgery.

Most commonly, the areas dietitians will find they need to counsel patients on before surgery include portion control, macronutrient and micronutrient composition of frequently chosen foods, skipping meals, and physical activity. Dietitians use various tools to help assess a patient's food and beverage intake, including the 24-hour recall and food frequency questionnaires. When counseling patients preoperatively, it is important to put the emphasis on how dietary and lifestyle changes positively affect long-term weight maintenance. Adhering to portion control before surgery will likely lead to preoperative weight loss, resulting in a lower weight 24 months after surgery. It will also help patients maintain their weight loss over the long term. Patients often state they are limited in food choices postoperatively. Developing a menu before surgery that includes a variety of soft proteins (e.g. low-fat dairy, beans, nut butters, fish), whole grains, fruits, vegetables, and healthy fats will empower patients to try new foods and recipes after surgery that are appropriate for the texture that they are able to tolerate. This will help stave off taste fatigue and provide a more nutritious diet as they are able to include more solid, textured foods [81]. Patients should also be working towards eliminating intake of sugar-sweetened beverages in the preoperative period and including mostly water and sugar-free beverages. While skipping any meal is discouraged, observational studies highlight that eating breakfast regularly can be an effective tool for weight management [82]. Regularly eating breakfast is associated with lower BMI in adults, and inclusion of whole grains, fruit, and low-fat dairy may be related to appetite control and blood glucose regulation, both contributing factors to obesity [83]. Patients often have the misconception that skipping breakfast will lead to eating fewer calories in the day, when in fact, skipping breakfast can lead to cravings of high-calorie foods later in the day [84]. Therefore, patients should be encouraged to include breakfast daily in order to better maintain weight loss after surgery.

Lastly, physical activity is consistently cited as a predictor of weight loss maintenance [85]. Despite being aware that physical activity has health benefits, barriers to exercise still remain. They include inability to self-motivate, lack of encouragement from family and friends, time constraints, low self-efficacy, fear of being injured, recent injury, and lack of resources (i.e. no sidewalks or parks in neighborhood) [86]. Overcoming barriers to exercise will likely take a team approach, including the dietitian, psychologist, and possibly a physical therapist. The patient should be encouraged to begin a rather simple exercise program that takes into account reservations about exercise and physical limitations. We often see that as patients begin exercise programs, they are hesitant and resistant; however, as their self-esteem improves and physical activity becomes less taxing on the body, they build upon the program and welcome the exercise. They report having more energy, looking forward to the time by themselves, and overall mood improvement. Walking for as little as 5 minutes per day can often lead to walking for 30 minutes 3-4 times per week over a 3-month span.

With regard to micronutrients, it is estimated that 2 billion people worldwide suffer from vitamin and mineral malnutrition despite adequate calorie intake. In the United States greater than 75% of people are taking in below the daily recommended value of vitamins A, D and E. Additionally, 50 to 75% of Americans are also not taking enough vitamin C [87]. These deficiencies are also seen in patients presenting for weight loss surgery. Obese patients are at increased risk for nutritional abnormalities in the preoperative setting; they have been found to be deficient in thiamine, folate, zinc, iron, ferritin, selenium, beta-carotene, magnesium, and vitamins A, B-12, C and D [88-92]. Vitamin D levels are also affected by latitude and this should also be taken into consideration when screening and supplementing these deficiencies. It is imperative to evaluate and supplement all nutritional deficits prior to surgery to prevent deficiencies which can be significantly more difficult to correct in the postoperative period. These micronutrients should be supplemented in the preoperative setting and monitored to ensure normal values before surgery. All patients undergo postoperative monitoring to guide supplementation after bariatric surgery with frequent regularly scheduled blood tests.

As bariatric surgery becomes a safer, more popular, and more accepted form of weight loss amongst health professionals, it is clear that a thorough preoperative nutritional assessment and consistent preoperative follow-up with the dietitian is essential for the patient to lose an appropriate amount of weight, avoid malnutrition, and to maintain the weight loss hopefully for life [93-95]. Whether the dietitian has 6 weeks or 6 months to work with the patient preoperatively, the main focus should be to build the foundation for a healthier lifestyle and better eating habits.

10. Psychological

The fight against obesity has many fronts. Simply reducing the capacity or absorption of the gastrointestinal tract will not have long lasting effects on weight if the psychosocial aspects of the disease are not addressed. An essential part of the preoperative evaluation is a psychological clearance [96]. The psychosocial and behavioral evaluation is geared to confirm the patient's ability to incorporate nutritional and behavioral changes before and after bariatric surgery. The psychological investigation is also used to identify cognitive, environmental, or psychiatric contraindications prior to surgery and to offer treatment for any disorders identified [97]. The obese adult population in the United States has been found to have higher incidence of major depression, bipolar disorder, generalized anxiety and panic disorder [98]. Intervening in these disease processes can enhance postoperative weight reduction; however, no definitive significant improvement in weight loss has been shown [53].

The interview consists of a standard psychological evaluation, evaluation of the patient's appropriateness for surgery, an assessment of eating behavior, stress, coping mechanisms, and social support. It is also used to confirm that the patient has the ability to consent and evaluate all the potential risks and possible benefits to surgery [96]. The psychosocial evaluation should be performed by a credentialed expert in psychology and behavior modification for all patients. Screening for eating disorders can involve using standardized assessments, see table 2 [96].

Mental illnesses and eating disorders identified during the screening process are not necessarily contraindications to surgery [99]. Their optimization is key for a durable and satisfying outcome. The bariatric surgeon should be aware that the patient may exhibit impression management during the preoperative psychological evaluation. This is done by purposefully

• Eating Disorder Examination Questionnaire
• Cleveland Clinic Behavioral Rating System
• Millon Behavioral Medicine Diagnostic (MBMD) (Pearson, San Antonio, Texas, USA)
• Alcohol Use Disorder Identification Test – Consumption (AUDIT-C)
• Beck Depression Inventory – II (BDI-II)
• Beck Anxiety Inventory (BAI)
• Multidimensional Health Locus of Control Scale
• Overeater's questionnaire

Table 2. Mental health assessment tools prior to weight loss surgery

minimizing psychological symptoms to receive a recommendation to proceed with surgery from the mental health professional. It is recommended that mental health professionals use measures to assess for impression management, as this will allow for proper preoperative treatment and minimize postoperative surprises [97].

11. Education

The process towards obtaining successful results after bariatric surgery begins during the preoperative period. The algorithm of care is a multi step process and requires full participation of both the practitioners and the patient. The ability to follow the plan of care and manage lifestyle changes required for successful weight loss depends on how well the patients are prepared prior to surgery. High patient satisfaction rating has been demonstrated after instituting a preoperative class for their bariatric patients [100]. Their class covered the following content: presurgery appointments, preparing for surgery, postoperative procedures, pain management, activity levels, wound care, nutrition, lifestyle changes and discharge instructions.

The ASMBS recommends having educational objectives and assessments throughout the preoperative period. It is suggested that the materials provided to the patients be at a sixth to eighth grade reading level to maximize comprehension [53]. Multimedia tools are also useful, however patients should be cautioned against using the internet as an information source as there is a high degree of bias, conflicting statements and out of date information [100]. The main goal of preoperative education is to provide information needed for informed consent, prepare the patient for the required lifestyle change and to establish realistic expectations regarding potential weight loss and quality of life improvements.

12. Functional status

A crucial component of the preoperative evaluation includes assessing the patient's ability to complete the activities of daily living. Bariatric patients have a high rate of comorbid conditions, some of which can cause physical limitation. Morbidly obese patients are also limited by their body habitus and weight related pain; this is especially true in the super morbidly obese patients. The limitations in mobility can impede on preoperative weight loss, cause psychological stress and limit access to care [101]. Preoperative functional status should be evaluated as it has been shown to be the strongest predictor for postoperative in hospital morbidity and mortality [102]. Our previously published data revealed that a completely dependent patient was 27 times more likely to experience mortality after bariatric surgery. The information gained from investigations into the patient's functional status is shared with the patient and risks, benefits and alternatives are discussed with the ability to offer a reasonable prognosis of the postoperative period.

Preoperative exercise has been found to reduce surgical complications, facilitate healing, achieve the mindset needed for positive behavior changes, and augment the rate of increased postoperative physical activity [103]. The ASMBS suggests exercise for 20 minutes, three to four days a week is sufficient to achieve these results [104]. Most bariatric surgery patients have sedentary lifestyles and low physical activity level. King and Bond describe a five step process to providing physical activity counseling to patients undergoing weight loss surgery [103].

The first step is to assess the patient's knowledge, beliefs and values regarding exercise along with prior and current levels of physical activity. The potential barriers successful implementation of a physical activity program should also be investigated at this point. Prior to beginning a physical activity program, the patients with current or a history of exercise intolerance should be referred to a cardiologist for proper exercise testing. Aside from cardiopulmonary restrictions to exercise, patients should be assessed for physical limitations such as sensory, balance and gait abnormalities – all of which can increase the risk of injury.

The second step is to advise the patient on the benefits of physical activity and develop realistic expectations. Strategies to increase safety and decrease barriers should be established. The patients should be taught how to gauge the level of intensity using the talk test or by measuring their own heart rate.

The thirds step is to come to a mutual agreement with the patient regarding their short, intermediate and long term physical activity goals. The goals should not be end results such as weight loss or maximal activity, but rather, specific goals regarding the frequency, duration and type of physical activity performed. It is recommended that the clinician set one goal that the patient has a high likelihood of achieving to boost confidence and encourage the patient to continue increasing their level of physical activity.

The fourth step is to assist the patient in achieving the goals by providing the patient printed materials and other resources that support self monitored physical activity. Such items include diaries, pedometers and a list of safe walking paths or fitness facilities. Patients who need a high level of encouragement or guidance, and those with significant barriers should be referred to professional personal trainers or other exercise professionals to achieve the best results.

The final step is to arrange for follow up and monitoring to answer questions and provide reinforcement. The patient and clinician should not be discouraged if the level of physical activity is not immediately increased after one meeting. It may take many visits for the patients to overcome their barriers and begin a physical activity plan. The healthcare provider should remain vigilant and provide continual counseling to the patient.

13. Conclusions

The preoperative evaluation of the bariatric surgery patient requires a multidisciplinary approach, ultimately coordinated by the surgeon. There are many details to which attention must be paid including medical, nutritional and psychological aspects in an effort to fully evaluate the patient as a whole. This multi faceted approach is one of the factors which have allowed bariatric surgery to become a safe and effective method for weight loss and comorbidity amelioration. These evaluations may reveal problems which should be addressed before surgery to ensure safety and success in the postoperative period. These assessments offer the best way to prepare and counsel a patient for these life altering operations and provide a reasonable basis of expectation on the part of the surgeon and the patient. Many of the learning points incorporated into the preoperative evaluation of bariatric patients can potentially be applied to other disciplines.

Author details

Gurdeep S. Matharoo[1], Erika Renick[1], John N. Afthinos[1], Tracey Straker[2] and Karen E. Gibbs[1*]

*Address all correspondence to: dockegibbs@gmail.com

1 Department of Surgery, Division of Minimally Invasive and Bariatric Surgery, Staten Island University Hospital, State University of New York, Brooklyn, USA

2 Department of Anesthesiology, Montefiore Medical Center, Albert Einstein College of Medicine, New York, USA

References

[1] National Institutes of Health. Gastrointestinal Surgery for Severe Obesity. NIH Consensus Statement Online. http://consensus.nih.gov/1991/1991gisurgeryobesity084html.htm. Accessed: November 2, 2013.

[2] Yermilov I, McGory ML, Shekelle PW. Appropriateness criteria for bariatric surgery: beyond the NIH guidelines. Obesity. 2009;17:1521-27.

[3] Fried M, Yumuk V, Oppert J, et al. Interdisciplinary European guidelines on metabolic and bariatric surgery. Obes Fact. 2013;6:449-68.

[4] Snijder MB, van Dam RM, Visser M, et al. What aspect of body fat are particularly hazardous and how do we measure them? Int J Epidemiol. 2006;35(1)83-92.

[5] Kasama K, Mui W, Lee WJ, et al. IFSO-APC Consensus Statements 2011. Obes Surg. 2012;22:677-84.

[6] Zalesin KC, Franklin BA, Miller WM, et al. Impact of obesity on cardiovascular disease. Med Clin N Am. 2011;95:919-937.

[7] Fleisher LA, Beckman JA, Brown KA, et al. ACC/AHA 2007 guidelines on perioperative cardiovascular evaluation and care for noncardiac surgery: executive summary: a report of the American College of Cardiology/American Heart Association Task Force on Practice Guidelines (Writing Committee to Revise the 2002 Guidelines on Perioperative Cardiovascular Evaluation for Noncardiac Surgery). Circulation. 2007;116:1971–1996.

[8] Mokdad, AH, Ford ES, Bowman BA, et al. Prevalence of obesity, diabetes and obesity-related health risk factors, 2001. JAMA. 2003;289;76-79.

[9] Padwal RS, Chang H, Klarenbach S, et al. Characteristic of the population eligible for and receiving publicly funded bariatric surgery in Canada. International Journal of Equity in Health. 2012; 11:54.

[10] DeMaria EJ, Portenier D, Wolfe L. Obesity surgery mortality risk score: proposal for a clnically useful score to predict mortality risk in patients undergoing gastric bypass. Surg Obes Relat Dis. 2007;3:134-40.

[11] Fleisher LA, Beckman JA, Brown KA, et al. 2009 ACCF/AHA focused update on perioperative beta blockade incorporated into the ACC/AHA 2007 guidelines on perioperative cardiovascular evaluation and care for noncardiac surgery: a report of the American College of Cardiology Foundation/American Heart Association Task Force on Practice Guidelines. J Am Coll Cardiol. 2009;54:e13–118.

[12] Katkhouda N, Mason RJ, Wu B, et al. Evaluation and treatment of patients with cardiac disease undergoing bariatric surgery. Surg Obes Relat Dis. 2012;8:634-40.

[13] Hansen CL, Woodhouse s, Kramer M. Effect of patient obesity on the accuracy of thallium-201 myocardial perfusion imaging. Am J Cardiol 2000;85:749-52

[14] Fihn SD, Gardin JM, Abrams J, et al. 2012 ACCF/AHA/ACP/AATS/PCNA/SCAI/STS guideline for the diagnosis and management of patients with stable ischemic heart disease: a report of the American College of Cardiology Foundation/American Heart Association Task Force on, American Association for Thoracic Surgery, Preventive Cardiovascular Nurses Association, Society for Cardiovascular Angiography and Interventions, and Society of Thoracic Surgeons. J Am Coll Cardiol 2012;60:e44–164.

[15] Darvish-Kazem S, Gandhi M, Marcucci M, et al. Perioperative management of antiplatelet therapy in patients with a coronary stent who need non-cardiac surgery: a systematic review of clinical practice guidelines. Chest. 2013 Aug 8. Epub ahead of print

[16] Khan MF, Movahed MR. Obesity cardiomyopathy and systolic function: obesity is not independently associated withdilated cardiomyopathy. Heart Fail Rev. 2013;18:207-17.

[17] Allman-Farinelli MA. Obesity and venous thrombosis: a review. Semin Thromb Hemost 2011;37:903-7.

[18] Mertens I, Van Gaal LF. Obesity, haemostasis and the fibrinolytic system. Obes Rev 2002;3:85-101.

[19] Kuruba R, Koche LS, Murr MM. Preoperative assessment and perioperative care of patients undergoing bariatric surgery. Med Clin N Am. 2007;339-51.

[20] The American Society for Metabolic and Bariatric Surgery Clinical Issues Committee. ASMBS updated position statement on prophylactic measures to reduce the risk of venous thromboembolism in bariatric surgery patients. Surg Obes Relat Dis. 2013;9:493-97

[21] Zierler BK. Ultrasonography and diagnosis of venous thromboembolism. Circulation. 2004;109:I9-I14.

[22] Prystowsky JB, Morasch MD, Eskandari, MK, et al. Prospective analysis of the incidence of deep venous thrombosis in bariatric surgery patients. Surgery. 2005;138:759-65.

[23] Westling A, Bergqvist D, Bostrom A. Incidence of deep venous thrombosis in patients undergoing obesity surgery. World J Surg. 2002;26:470-3.

[24] Gargiulo NJ 3rd, Veith FJ, Lipsitz EC, et al. The incidence of pulmonary embolism in open versus laparoscopic gastric bypass. Ann Vasc Surg. 2007;21:556-9.

[25] Gargiulo NJ 3rd, O'Connor DJ, Veith FJ, et al. Long-term outcome of inferior vena cava filter placement in patients undergoing gastric bypass. Ann Vasc Surg. 2010;24:946-9.

[26] Birkmeyer NJO, Share D, Baser O, et al. Preoperative placement of inferior vena cava filters and outcomes after gastric bypass surgery. Ann Surg. 2010;252:313-8.

[27] U.S. Food and Drug Administration. Removing retrievable inferior vena cava filters: initial communication. August 9, 2010. Available at: http://www.fda.gov/MedicalDevices/Safety/AlertsandNotices/ucm221676.htm. Accessed November 2, 2013.

[28] Birkmeyer NJ, Finks JF, English WJ, et al. Risk and benefits of prophylactic inferior vena cava filters in patients undergoing bariatric surgery. Journal of Hospital Medicine. 2013;8:173-77.

[29] Hsu P, Basu CB, Venturi M, et al. Venous thromboembolism prophylaxis. Semin Plast Surg. 2006;20(4):225-32.

[30] Becattini C, Agnelli G, Manina G, et al. Venous thromboembolism after laparoscopic bariatric surgery for morbid obesity: clinical burden and preventions. Surg Obes Relat Dis 2012;8:108-15

[31] Kemkes-Matthes B. Hirudin for prophylaxis and treatment of deep vein thrombosis. Semin Thromb Hemost. 2002;28(5):455-8.

[32] Mosen DM, Schatz M, Magid DJ, et al. The relationship between obesity and asthma severity and control in adults. J Allergy Clin Immunol. 2008;122:507-11. e6.

[33] Beuther DA, Sutherland ER. Overweight, obesity and incident asthma: a meta-analysis of prospective epidemiologic studies. Am J Respir Crit Care Med. 2007;175:661-6

[34] Hamoui N, Anthone G, Crookes PF. The value of pulmonary function testing prior to bariatric surgery. Obes Surg. 2006;16:1570-73

[35] van Huisstede A, Biter LU, Luitwieler R, et al. Pulmonary function testing and complications of laparoscopic bariatric surgery. Obes Surg. 2013;23:1596-1603.

[36] Masoomi H, Reavis KM, Smith BR, et al. Risk factors for acutre respiratory failure in bariatric surgery: data from the Nationwide Inpatient Sample, 2006 – 2008. Surg Obes Relat Dis. 2013;9:277-83.

[37] Marchini JFM, Souza FLN, Schmidt A, et al. Low educational status, smoking, and multidisciplinary team experience predict hospital length of stay after bariatric surgery. Nutr Metab Insights. 2012;5:71-6.

[38] Azagury DE, Abu Dayyeh BK, Greenwalt IT, et al. Marginal ulceration after roux-en-y gastric bypass surgery: characteristics, risk factors, treatment, and outcomes. Endoscopy. 2011;43:950-4.

[39] Fawcett A, Shembekar M, Church JS, et al. Smoking, hypertension, and colonic anastomotic healing; a combinded clinical and histopathological study. Gut. 1996;38:714-8.

[40] ASMBS Clinical Issues Committee et al. Perioperative management of obstructive sleep apnea. Surg Obes Relat Dis. 2012;8:e27-e32.

[41] Berry RB; Budhiraja R; Gottlieb DJ; et al. Rules for scoring respiratory events in sleep: update of the 2007 AASM Manual for the Scoring of Sleep and Associated Events. J Clin Sleep Med 2012;8(5):597-619.

[42] Ramirez A, Lalor PF, Szomstein S, et al. Continuous positive airway pressure in immediate postoperative period after laparoscopic roux-en-y gastric bypass: is it safe? Surg Obes Relat Dis. 2009;5:544-6.

[43] Chau EHL, Lam D, Wong J, et al. Obesity hypoventilation syndrome a review of epidemiology, pathophysiology, and perioperative considerations. Anesthesiology. 2012;117:118-205

[44] Khan A, King WB, Patterson EJ, et al. Assessment of obstructive sleep apnea in adults undergoing bariatric surgery in the Longitudinal Assessment of Bariatric Surgery-2 (LABS-2) study. J Clin Sleep Med. 2013;9(1):21-9.

[45] Ogunnaike B, Jones SB, Jones DB, et al. Anesthetic considerations for bariatric surgery. Anesth Analg. 2002;95:1793-1805.

[46] Kheterpal S, Han R, Tremper KK, et al. Incidence and predictors of difficult mask ventilation. Anesthesiology 2006;105(5):885-891.

[47] Neligan PJ, Porter s, Max B, et al. Obstructive sleep apnea is not a risk factor for difficult intubation in morbidly obese patients. Anesth Analg. 2009;109(4):1182-6.

[48] Lebowitz PW, Shay H, Straker T,et al. Shoulder and head elevation improves laryngoscopic view for tracheal intubation in non obese as well as obese individuals. J Clin Anesth. 2012;24(2):104-8.

[49] Brodsky JB, Lemmens JM, Brock-Utne JG, et al. Morbid obesity and tracheal intubation. Anesth Analg. 2002;94(3):732-736.

[50] Vaugh RW, Bauer S, Wise L. Volume and pH of gastric juice in obese patients. Anesthesiology 1975;43(6):686-689.

[51] Apfelbaum JL, Hagberg CA, Caplan RA, et al. Practice guidelines for management of the difficult airway: an updated report by the American Society of Anesthesiologists Task Force on Management of the Difficult Airway. Anesthesiology. 2013;118(2): 251-70

[52] Anesthesiology News – Guide to Airway Management. Airway management in the patient undergoing bariatric surgery. Available at http://www.anesthesiologynews.com/download/Bariatric_ANGAM09_WM.pdf. Accesibility verified: November 4, 2013.

[53] Mechanick JI, Youdim A, Jones DB, et al. Clinical practice guidelines for the perioperative nutritional, metabolic, and nonsurgical support of the bariatric surgery patient--2013 update: cosponsored by American Association of Clinical Endocrinologists, the Obesity Society, and American Society for Metabolic & Bariatric Surgery. Surg Obes Relat Dis. 2013;9:159-91.

[54] Jankovic D, Wolf P, Anderwald C, et al. Prevalence of endocrine disorders in morbidly obese patients and the effects of bariatric surgery on endocrine and metabolic parameters. Obes Surg. 2012;22:62-69.

[55] Perna M, Romagnuolo J, Morgan K et al. Preoperative hemoglobin A1c and postoperative glucose control in outcomes after gastric bypass for obesity. Surg Obes Relat Dis. 2012;6:686-90.

[56] National Institutes of Health. The Practical Guide: Identification, Evaluation, and Treatment of Overweight and Obesity in Adults. http://www.nhlbi.nih.gov/guidelines/obesity/prctgd_b.pdf. Accessed 10/26/2013.

[57] Hampel H, Abraham NS, El-Serag HB. Meta-analysis: obesity and the risk for gastroesophageal reflux disease and its complications. Ann Intern Med. 2005;143(3):199-211.

[58] Greenwald D. Preoperative gastrointestinal assessment before bariatric surgery. Gastroenterol Clin N Am. 2010;19;81-6.

[59] Verma S, Sharma D, Kanwar P, et al. Prevalence of Helicobacter pylori infection in bariatric patients: a histologic assessment. Surg Obes Relat Dis. 2013;9(5):679-85.

[60] Rawlins L, Rawlins MP, Brown CC, Schumacher DL. Effect of Helicobacter pylori on marginal ulcer and stomal stenosis after roux-en-y gastric bypass. Surg Obes Relat Dis. 2013;9:760-4.

[61] World Health Organization. Global Burden of Disease – 2004 Update. Geneva, Switzerland. WHO Press; 2008

[62] Che F, Nguyen B, Cohen A, et al. Prevalence of hiatal hernia in the morbidly obese. Surg Obes Relat Dis. 2013 Apr 19. Epub ahead of print

[63] Fris RJ. Preoperative low energy diet diminishes liver size. Obesity Surg. 2004;14:1165-70.

[64] Edholm D, Kullberg J, Haenni A, et al. Preoperative 4-week low-calorie diet reduces liver volume and intrahepatic fat and facilitates laparoscopic gastric bypass in morbidly obese. Obes Surg. 2011;21:345-50.

[65] Guadalajara H, Sanz Boro R, Pascual I, et al. Is prophylactic cholecystectomy useful in obese patients undergoing gastric bypass? Obes Surg. 2006;16(7):883-5.

[66] Liem RK, Niloff PH. Prophylactic Cholecystectomy with open gastric bypass operation. Obes Surg. 2004;14:763-5.

[67] Hamad GG, Ikramuddin S, Gourash WF, et al. Elective cholecystectomy during laparoscopic gastric bypass: is it worth the wait? Obesity Surg. 2003;13:76-81.

[68] D'Hondt M, Sergeant G, Deylgat B, et al. Prophylactic cholecystectomy, a mandatory step in morbidly obese patients undergoing laparoscopic Roux-en-Y gastric bypass? J Gastrointest Surg. 2011;15:1532-36.

[69] Biesemeier CK, Garland J, eds. ADA Pocket Guide to Bariatric Surgery. Chicago, IL: American Dietetic Association; 2009.

[70] Aills L, Blankenship J, Buffington C, et al. ASMBS allied health nutritional guidelines for the surgical weight loss patient. Surg Obes Relat Dis. 2008;4(5 Suppl):S73-S108.

[71] National Eating Disorders Association. Factors that may contribute to eating disorders page. Accessibility verified: http://www.nationaleatingdisorders.org/contributing-factors-prevention. Accessed November 1, 2013.

[72] Beckman LM, Beckman TR, Earthman CP. Changes in gastrointestinal hormones and leptin after Roux-en-Y gastric bypass procedure: a review. J Am diet Assoc. 2010;110(4):571-84.

[73] Karpyn A, Young C, Weiss S. Reestablishing healthy food retail: changing the landscape of food deserts. Child Obes. 2012;8(1):28-30.

[74] Herichova I. Changes of physiological functions induced by shift work. Endocr Regul. 2013;47(3):159-70.

[75] Geliebter A, Gluck ME, Tanowitz M, et al. Work-shift period and weight change. Nutrition. 2000;16(1):27-29.

[76] McAlpine DE, Frisch MJ, Romes ES, et al. Bariatric surgery: a primer for eating disorder professionals. Eur Eat Disord Rev. 2010;18(4):304-17.

[77] Sandberg RM, Dahl JK, Vedul-Kjelsas E, et al. Health-related quality of life in obese presurgery patients with and without binge eating disorder, and subdiagnostic binge eating disorders. J Obes. 2013;2013:878310.

[78] Snyder, AG. Psychological assessment of the patient undergoing bariatric surgery. Oschner J. 2009;9(3):144-8.

[79] Kinzl JF, Schrattenecker M, Traweger C, et al. Psychosocial predictors of weight loss after bariatric surgery. Obes Surg. 2006;16(12):1609-14.

[80] Chesler BE. Emotional eating: a virtually untreated risk factor for outcome following bariatric surgery. ScienteificWorldJournal. 2012;2012:365961.

[81] Thomas J, Gizis F, Marcus E. Food selections of Roux-en-Y gastric bypass patients up to 2.5 years postsurgery. J Am Diet Assoc. 2010;110(4):608-12.

[82] Timlin MT, Pereira MA. Breakfast frequency and quality in the etiology of obesity and chronic diseases. Nutr Rev. 2007;65(6 Pt 1): 268-81.

[83] Pereira MA, Erickson E, McKee P. Breakfast frequency and quality may affect glycemia in adults and children. J Nutr. 2011;141(1):163-8.

[84] Goldstone AP, Prechtl de Hernandez CG, Beaver JD, et al. Fasting biases brain reward systems towards high-calorie foods. Eur J Neurosci. 2009;30(8):1625-35.

[85] National Weight Control Registry. NWCR facts page. Available at: http://www.nwcr.ws/Research/default.htm. Accessibility verified: November 1, 2013.

[86] Centers for Disease Control. Overcoming barriers to physical activity page. Available at: http://www.cdc.gov/physicalactivity/everyone/getactive/barriers.html. Accessibility verified: November 1, 2013.

[87] Nicoletti CF, Lima TP, Donadelli SP, et al. New look at nutritional care for obese patient candidates for bariatric surgery. Surg Obes Relat Dis. 2013;9:520-5.

[88] Schweiger C, Weiss R, Berry E, Keidar A. Nutritional deficiencies in bariatric surgery candidates. Obes Surg. 2010;20:193-7.

[89] Germmel K, Santry HP, Prachand VN, Alverdy JC. Vitamin D deficiency in perioperative bariatric surgery patients. Surg Obes Relat Dis. 2009;5:54-9.

[90] Hoeft B, Weber P, Eggerdorfer M. Micronutrient – a global perspective on intake, health benefits and economics. Int J Nutr Res. 2012;82(5):312-20.

[91] Kaidar-Person O, Person B, Szomstein S, et al. Nutritional deficiencies in morbidly obese patients: a new form of malnutrition? Part A: vitamins. Obes Surg. 2008;18(7): 870-6

[92] Kaidar-Person O, Person B, Szomstein S, et al. Nutritional deficiencies in morbidly obese patients: a new form of malnutrition? Part B: minerals. Obes Surg. 2008;18(8): 1028-34.

[93] Kulick D, Hark L, Deen D. The bariatric surgery patient: a growing role for registered dietitians. J Am Diet Assoc. 2010;110(4):593-9.

[94] Kushner RF, Neff LM. Bariatric surgery: a key role for registered dietitians. J Am Diet Assoc. 2010;110(4):524-6.

[95] Van Horn, L. The registered dietitian's role in treating bariatric surgery patients. J AM Diet Assoc. 2010;110(4):497.

[96] Heinberg LJ, Ashton K, Windover A. Moving beyond dichotomous psychological evaluation: the Cleveland Clinic Behavioral Rating System for weight loss surgery. Surg Obes Relat Dis. 2010;6:185-90.

[97] Ambwani S, Boeka AG, Brown JD, et al. Socially desirable responding by bariatric surgery candidates during psychological assessment. Surg Obes Relat Dis. 2013;9:300-5.

[98] Simon GE, Von Korff M, Saunders K, et al. Association between obesity and psychiatric disorders in the US adult population. Arch Gen Psychiatry. 2006;63:824-30.

[99] Greenberg I, Sogg S, Perna FM. Behavioral and psychological care in weight loss surgery: Best practice update. Obesity. 2009;17:880-4.

[100] Goldstein N, Hadidi N. Impact of bariatric preoperative education on patient knowledge and satisfaction with overall hospital experience. Bariatr Nurs Surg Patient Care. 2010;5:137-44.

[101] Kalarchian MA, Marcus MD, Levine MD, et al. Psychiatric disorders among bariatric surgery candidates: relationship to obesity and functional health status. Am j Psychiatry 2007; 164:328-34.

[102] Khan MA, Grinberg R, Johnson S, et al. Perioperative risk factors for 30-day mortality after bariatric surgery: is functional status important? Surg Endosc. 2013;27:1772-7.

[103] King WC, Bond DS. The importance of preoperative and postoperative physical activity counseling in bariatric surgery. Exerc Sport Sci Rev. 2013;41(1):26-35.

[104] American Society for Metabolic and Bariatric Surgery. ASMBS Public and Professional Education Committee. Bariatric Surgery: Postoperative Concerns. http://s3.amazonaws.com/publicASMBS/GuidelinesStatements/Guidelines/asbs_bspc.pdf. Accessed 10/28/2013.

Chapter 2

Theoretical Bases and Dietary Approach of Bariatric Patients

Patrícia Fátima Sousa Novais, Flávia Andreia Marin,
Alex Harley Crisp, Irineu Rasera Junior,
Celso Vieira de Souza Leite and
Maria Rita Marques de Oliveira

Additional information is available at the end of the chapter

http://dx.doi.org/10.5772/58636

1. Introduction

Obesity ultimately results from an unbalance between the intake and oxidation of the energy obtained from foods, and its treatments are based on correcting this unbalance by basically restricting energy intake. Consequently, food intake is the center of attention when the subject is obesity, either as an etiological, protection, or even therapeutic factor.

The inability of severely obese individuals to reduce or maintain their body weight using traditional methods makes them candidates to bariatric surgery, which is admittedly an effective method to reduce body weight significantly and obesity-associated morbidities. Bariatric surgery involves anatomic and physiological changes in the gastrointestinal tract that promote energy restriction, essential for weight loss, but also the restriction of many essential dietary nutrients. In addition to the anatomic aspects, bariatric surgery decreases appetite and increases postprandial satiety, possibly because of its effect on the secretion of hormones that regulate these systems (Kohli, Stefater e Inge, 2011).

In addition to reducing body weight significantly, bariatric surgery also decreases some systemic inflammation markers (Chen et al., 2009; Miller et al., 2011), improves insulin sensitivity, promoting remission of type 2 diabetes (T2D), and lowers high blood pressure, among others.

Although bariatric surgery is associated with better quality of life, nutritional deficiencies may occur after surgery because of the dramatically reduced food intake and/or micronutrient

INTECH
open science | open minds

© 2014 The Author(s). Licensee InTech. This chapter is distributed under the terms of the Creative Commons Attribution License (http://creativecommons.org/licenses/by/3.0), which permits unrestricted use, distribution, and reproduction in any medium, provided the original work is properly cited.

absorption. Unmonitored postoperative patients may develop severe malnutrition (Dodell et al., 2012). The literature has often reported deficiencies of vitamin B complex, iron, folic acid, vitamin D, and calcium (Saltzman e Karl, 2013). These deficiencies may cause neurological symptoms, osteopenia, and anemia.

Hence, the nutritional approach of the bariatric patient, which began when the patient was in line for surgery and continued after surgery, is one of the most important themes of the interdisciplinary care of obese patients. The objective of this chapter is to review the theoretical bases for the nutritional approach of bariatric patients, the instruments for assessing food intake, and the nutritional recommendations, both preoperatively, when the patient is preparing for surgery, and postoperatively, during follow-up. The chapter also includes practical examples.

2. The nutrition process after bariatric surgery

The surgeries used for treating severe obesity include restrictive surgeries that limit food intake, such as vertical banded gastroplasty (VBG), adjustable gastric band (AGB), and sleeve gastrectomy (SG); and mixed surgeries that combine food intake restriction with nutrient malabsorption, such as Roux-en-Y gastric bypass (RYGB) and biliopancreatic diversion (BPD) with duodenal switch (BPD-DS) (Pories, 2008).

The implications of surgery on nutritional status stem specifically from the types of anatomic and physiological changes the surgery makes. The main macro-and micronutrient absorption sites reflect the dimension of the nutritional impairment, especially in the long run, and the possible nutritional complications promoted by bariatric surgery, a situation that should be prevented with appropriate monitoring and supplementation.

In restrictive surgeries, nutritional deficiencies are associated with inadequate food intake, while in malabsorptive interventions, deficiencies are more associated with the hindrance of nutrient digestion and absorption. In summary, the energy deficit caused by low macronutrient intake and/or absorption is accompanied by inadequate intake of essential nutrients.

The small intestine, target of the bypasses associated with malabsorptive techniques, is where most of food digestion and absorption occurs. The absorption of iron (Fe), calcium (Ca), zinc (Zn), selenium (Se), copper (Cu), and some water-soluble vitamins, such as vitamin C, thiamin (B_1), and riboflavin (B_2) occurs in the duodenum; the absorption of Fe, Zn, chromium, amino acids, peptides, carbohydrates, lipids, the fat-soluble vitamins A, D, E, and K, and most of the water-soluble vitamins occurs in the jejunum; and the absorption of amino acids, peptides, lipids, fat-soluble vitamins, magnesium, vitamin B_{12}, and folic acid occurs in the ileum. Generally, the most common micronutrient deficiencies after bariatric surgery are Fe, Ca, vitamin D, vitamin B_{12}, folic acid, and Zn (Bloomberg et al., 2005).

In BPD associated with gastrectomy, mostly a malabsorptive mixed surgery, nutrient malabsorption is even greater, causing massive nutrient loss. Nutrient malabsorption is one of the factors that explain weight loss promoted by malabsorptive techniques, but techniques that are mostly malabsorptive reduce the intestinal absorption capacity significantly. BPD, for instance, decreases protein absorption by 25% and fat absorption by 72%, impairing the absorption of fat-soluble vitamins (Aills et al., 2008). BPD-DS lowers the serum concentration of thiamin in the first few months after surgery and of vitamins A and D one year after surgery more than RYGB does (Aasheim et al., 2009).

Today the main type of bariatric surgery done globally is RYGB, which reduces gastric capacity and causes a small degree of malabsorption as it bypasses the duodenum and a small part of the jejunum, namely, 30 centimeters of the proximal jejunum. Nevertheless, the bypassed segments can influence the absorption of proteins and some water-soluble vitamins, namely vitamins C, B_1, B_2, B_6, and folic acid, absorbed in the proximal jejunum. Fat-soluble vitamins that require lipids to be absorbed may also be affected. Hence, mineral deficiencies in RYGB, such as Fe, Ca, and Zn stem from proximal small intestine bypass, specifically from duodenum bypass.

Vitamin and mineral deficiencies at first are asymptomatic or present unspecific symptoms. Laboratory tests are necessary to monitor and avoid the development of postoperative nutritional and clinical complications. Nutritional deficiencies found one year after surgery included Fe (51%), Ca and vitamin D (47%), folic acid (39%), and Zn (12%) (Gasteyger et al., 2008).

- **Calcium and vitamin D**

Calcium and vitamin D deficiencies in obese patients in line for bariatric surgery are common, as well as high parathyroid hormone (PTH). Assessment of calcium metabolism should include measuring serum PTH, total calcium, phosphorus, 25-hydroxycholecalciferol, and the calcium present in 24 hours of urine. The normal levels of vitamin D, 25-hydroxycholecalciferol, or 25(OH)D range from 30 to 80 ng/mL. Vitamin D insufficiency occurs when these levels are below 30 but above 20ng/mL and deficiency when below 20ng/mL. The prevalences of vitamin D deficiency before and one year after RYGB were 86% and 70%, respectively (Signori et al., 2010). This deficiency may stem from inadequate intake and higher calcium and vitamin D requirements after surgery since the main calcium absorption sites are located in the bypassed intestinal section. Calcium, PTH, and vitamin D levels should be normalized before and after surgery to avoid bone loss.

In a sample of 30 female RYGB patients assessed eight years ago, Duran de Campos et al. (2008) found osteopenia (67%), osteoporosis (13%), low urine calcium (70%), vitamin D deficiency (90%), and high markers of bone metabolism, namely high PTH (54%) and high alkaline phosphatase (57%). Their mean calcium intake was roughly 50% of their daily requirement (1000mg), suggesting that bariatric patients should be encouraged to consume an adequate amount of calcium.

- **Iron**

Iron deficiency is the main cause of anemia in bariatric patients. However, other nutrients associated with anemia are also malabsorbed, such as proteins and micronutrients required for iron metabolism and erythropoiesis, such as zinc, copper, folic acid, vitamin B_{12}, and vitamin A. Specifically, iron deficiency may stem from three events: 1) less dietary iron, especially heme iron present in meats; 2) less hydrochloric acid because of the stomach bypass, which reduces the dissolution of iron salts; and 3) duodenum bypass, given that the duodenum is the main site of iron absorption (Ruz et al. 2009).

The prevalence of anemia in bariatric patients varies according to time elapsed since surgery, type of surgery, and sex, with women of childbearing age being more vulnerable. In a prospective study of 1125 RYGB patients of which 999 were females, Drygalski et al. (2011) found a prevalence of anemia of 12% six months after surgery, which increased to 21% eighteen months after surgery and 23% one to two years after surgery. Six months after surgery, the prevalence of anemia in menopausal women was 6% against 16% in premenopausal women.

- **Vitamin B12**

The absorption of vitamin B12 is also impaired by gastric restriction, a procedure performed in restrictive, mixed, and mostly malabsorptive surgeries. Although the absorption of vitamin B12 occurs in the terminal ileum, B12 can only be absorbed when bound to an intrinsic factor, a glycoprotein produced by parietal cells, in the presence of hydrochloric acid and pepsin. These molecular interactions usually occur in the distal stomach and duodenum, and RYGB bypasses both (Flancbaum et al., 2006).

Vitamin B12 deficiency is common: 33-40% of the patients develop it one year after RYGB (Brolin et al., 2002). A study found that RYGB patients taking conventional nutrient supplementation still developed B12 deficiency and required further supplementation. The most common deficiency was of vitamin B12: 62% and 80% of the patients had it one and two years after surgery, respectively. A combined deficiency of vitamin B_{12} and folic acid may cause megaloblastic anemia (Heber et al., 2010). Other studies have reported that conventional supplementation is enough to prevent folic acid deficiency. In addition to the dosages present in multivitamins, our patients take a quarterly injection of Citoneurin 5000UI, rich in B complex.

- **Generality**

Deficiencies present preoperatively, such as iron (44%), vitamin D (68%), and thiamin (29%) deficiencies (Flancbaum et al., 2006), may worsen after surgery, but few studies have investigated how preoperative deficiencies relate to postoperative nutritional complications, another theme requiring further investigation. Another particularity that deserves attention regards iron, since preoperative deficiency may not be exclusively nutritional: the inflammation associated with obesity hinders the regulation of iron metabolism, promoting the development of functional iron deficiency. Iron homeostasis is regulated by hepcidin, a circulating peptide hormone produced mainly by hepatocytes but also by adipocytes, which acts as a negative regulator of iron metabolism (Bekri et al., 2006). Studies grouping these two situations, preoperative functional deficiency and postoperative iron levels, may clarify current perspectives and establish new ones on iron supplementation.

The significant changes made by bariatric surgery reduce energy intake and intestinal absorptive capacity, factors that contribute to weight loss. In addition to the anatomic and physiological changes, bariatric surgery promotes hormonal changes, such as reducing ghrelin production in the fundus of the stomach (an important endogenous orexigenic) and increasing intestinal hormones, namely peptide YY, glucagon-like peptide-1 (GLP-1), and gastric inhibitory polypeptide (GIP). The presence of poorly digested food in the distal small intestine after RYGB and BPD seem to stimulate the production of gut hormones, increasing incretins, GLP-1, and GIP, which help to control postoperative weight and glycemia (Rodieux et al., 2008). GLP-1 has a significant postprandial incretin effect, affecting insulin secretion, modulating appetite and gastric emptying, and eventually impacting the capture of glucose by tissues. Although some studies emphasize the role of lower serum ghrelin and higher incretin on satiety and weight control, other studies have not ultimately confirmed that hunger, satiety, and weight loss are related to these hormonal changes, so more studies are needed (Heber et al., 2010).

3. The nutritional needs of obese and ex-obese individuals

Although obesity is caused by an intake of macronutrients in excess of the body's requirement, certain nutrient deficiencies are often present in obese individuals. High intake of processed, energy-dense foods of usually poor nutritional value contributes significantly to micronutrient deficiencies. Additionally, an increase in adiposity and consequent oxidative stress may reduce the levels of some fat-soluble vitamins and nonenzymatic antioxidants. As a matter of fact, population data have shown that micronutrient inadequacy is greater among overweight and obese adults (Kimmons et al., 2006).

Patients in the waiting line for bariatric surgery have a high to moderate prevalence of the following deficiencies: calcium (Jastrzębska-Mierzyńska et al., 2012), folic acid (Schweiger et al., 2010; Jastrzębska-Mierzyńska et al., 2012; de Luis et al., 2013), iron (Flancbaum et al., 2006; Schweiger et al., 2010; Jastrzębska-Mierzyńska et al., 2012), vitamin A (Nicoletti et al., 2013), vitamin C (Aasheim et al., 2008; Nicoletti et al., 2013), vitamin E (Aasheim et al., 2008), vitamin B_1 (Flancbaum et al., 2006), vitamin B_6 (Aasheim et al., 2008; Moizé et al., 2011;), vitamin B_{12} (Ernst et al., 2009; Nicoletti et al., 2013), magnesium (Moizé et al., 2011; Nicoletti et al., 2013), copper (de Luis et al., 2013), and zinc (Ernst et al., 2009; de Luis et al., 2013). The prevalence of anemia is also moderate to high (Flancbaum et al., 2006; Schweiger et al., 2010; Moizé et al., 2011). Finally, vitamin D deficiency has been the most often reported deficiency (Flancbaum et al., 2006; Carlin et al., 2006; Aasheim et al., 2008; Toh, Zarshenas, Jorgensen, 2009; Gammel et al., 2009; Fish et al., 2010; Casagrande et al., 2010; Ducloux et al., 2011; Moizé et al., 2011; Jastrzębska-Mierzyńska et al., 2012; de Luis et al., 2013; Censani et al., 2013).

Vitamin D is a fat-soluble vitamin with hormonal functions. It acts on many tissues especially through nuclear and membrane receptors. Evidence shows that vitamin D is essential for bone mineralization and acts on the pancreas, immune system, and nervous system, among others. Low vitamin D in obese individuals may be related to low dietary bioavailability, inadequate sunlight exposure, and even sequestration by adipose tissue (Brouwer et al., 1998). Some studies report a low to moderate inverse correlation between serum vitamin D and body mass index (Parikn et al., 2004; Carlin et al., 2005; McGil et al., 2008; Cimbek et al., 2012; Taheri et al., 2012).

The prevalences of micronutrient deficiencies vary between studies (Flancbaum et al., 2006; Carlin et al., 2006; Aasheim et al., 2008; Toh, Zarshenas, Jorgensen, 2009; Gammel et al., 2009; Fish et al., 2010; Casagrande et al., 2010; Ducloux et al., 2011; Moizé et al., 2011; Jastrzębska-Mierzyńska et al., 2012; de Luis et al., 2013; Censani et al., 2013). These differences may stem from different food habits, which vary between cities, states, and countries. Therefore, nutritional assessment by laboratory tests and food surveys is strongly recommended to detect nutritional insufficiencies early and make the necessary nutritional interventions. Symptoms caused by undetected preexisting deficiencies may become worse during the postoperative period. Since biochemical tests are expensive, Mechanick et al., (2013) suggest starting micronutrient supplementation in the preoperative period.

Gastric surgery is essential for promoting energy intake restriction and consequently, energy deficit and weight loss. Nonetheless, this procedure may induce strong aversion to certain foods, malnutrition, and specific micronutrient deficiencies. Recently, the American Association of Clinical Endocrinologists, The Obesity Society and the American Society for Metabolic & Bariatric Surgery (Mechanick et al., 2013) published the nutritional requirements of ex-obese bariatric patients. In summary, these individuals should take multivitamin and multimineral supplements that help them to meet their daily requirements of the main micronutrients (elemental calcium: 1200-1500 mg; vitamin D: 3000 IU; vitamin B_{12}: 1000 mcg; folic acid: 400 μg; iron: 45-60 mg) and protein (1.5 grams (60g/d) per kilogram of body weight).

4. Food intake assessment

Determining food intake is a constant challenge for the science and practice of nutrition and dietetics. Food surveys indirectly assess nutritional status. They are always under scrutiny because of their limited ability to measure energy and nutrient intakes. Quantitative and qualitative food intake can be determined by different methods, such as recalls, in which individuals remember the foods they ate. The most important of these retrospective methods are the food frequency questionnaire (FFQ) and the 24-hour recall (24HR). Food intake may also be investigated prospectively by asking individuals to write down the foods they eat in a food diary or record (FD) the moment they eat them (Gibson, 2005; Anjos et al., 2009).

The food intake survey of choice depends on the study objectives and population, but administering a single 24HR or FD to assess habitual food intake is not recommended, not even for obese individuals. Intraindividual variations, that is, daily variations in food intake, occur, so at least two surveys should be administered on alternate days. Some studies recommend three 24HR or FD administered on alternate days, including a weekend day (Johnson, 2002), which allows statistical adjustment of the variances of the study days' mean. Some factors may distort food intake data, such as the interviewer's skill, interviewee's memory, and interview's environment. Moreover, the assessment itself may affect an individual's intake pattern and consequently, information quality. Nutrient intake estimates may also err because of the use of standard recipes and data variation in food composition tables (Dodd et al., 2006).

The food intake assessment of obese patients consists of many challenges, such as obtaining reliable information, identifying underreporting, correctly estimating energy and nutrient requirements, and establishing the appropriate interventions (Anjos et al., 2009).

A common finding in studies that assess the food intake of obese individuals is low energy intake, which may stem from food intake underreporting and/or physical activity overreporting (Macdiarmid; Blundell, 1998; Lichtman et al., 1992). Individual characteristics associated with underreporting include being older, female, and physically inactive; having low social and educational levels; restricting foods; experiencing emotional changes (Abbot et al., 2008; Macdiarmid; Blundell, 1998); and especially, having a high body mass index, that is, being overweight or obese (Rennie, Coward, Jebb, 2007; Scagliusi et al, 2009).

The classification of individuals as underreporters is based on the premise that individuals in energy balance, that is, whose weights are constant, have equivalent energy intake and expenditure (Goldberg et al., 1991; Trabulsi; Schoeller, 2001). Energy intake determined by quantitative survey can be confirmed by doubly labeled water (DLW), which accurately measures total energy expenditure (TEE) (Schoeller, 1999). The energy intake reported in food intake assessments is usually much lower than the actual energy intake (Black, Cole, 2001).

A review of DLW and calorimetry studies treated the intra-and interindividual energy intake variations statistically to establish the cutoff points that identify the lowest, plausible energy intake levels and expressed them as multiples of the resting energy expenditure (REE) (Goldberg et al., 1991). The TEE:REE ratio is known as the physical activity level (PAL). In energy balance, reported energy intake (EIrep) divided by REE should be equal to the TEE divided by REE, that is, EIrep:REE=TEE:REE or EIrep:REE=PAL. Many adjustments have been proposed to maximize the sensitivity and specificity of the cutoff point. Different studies have replaced variables of the Goldberg's equation, one at a time, by constants (Black, 2000), especially PAL, sample size, and number of food intake assessments (Black et al., 1991; Black, 2000; Goldberg et al., 1991; Abbot et al., 2008). Our research group Quesada (2011) used the Goldberg's equation in six different ways to classify the underreporting of 100 morbidly obese women. The prevalence of underreporting varied significantly, from 43% to 92%. This difference stemmed mainly from the intraindividual variations of the study sample, namely PAL and sample size, which minimized the underreporting interpretation error when used in the equation.

Nowadays studies tend to investigate food pattern, as opposed to individual nutrients, to establish relationships between diet and the health statuses of intragroup individuals (Hu, 2002). Dietary pattern analysis characterizes the eating behavior of population groups, elucidating the association between diet and health and/or other factors (Moeller et al., 2007). Dietary patterns characterized by the intake of fruits, vegetables, whole grains, fish, and poultry have been associated with a high intake of micronutrients and with selected biomarkers of dietary exposure and disease risk in the expected direction (Kant, 2004).

The association of one or a few nutrients with a given disease has conceptual and methodological limitations (Hu, 2002). These limitations are evidenced by the fact that they do not take into account the complex synergy between dietary nutrients, the cumulative effects and multiple nutrients that compose dietary patterns, the statistical significance that a wide range of chemical elements or foods can produce, and the relationship of association between the intake of certain nutrients and dietary patterns (Moeller et al., 2007). Hence, dietary pattern analysis has emerged as an alternative and complementary approach in nutritional epidemiological studies that evidence the relationship between the overall diet and the risk of chronic diseases (Hu, 2002).

Multivariate statistical analyses have been used for defining dietary patterns. Factor analysis, which includes both principal component analysis (PCA) and factorial analysis, is a multivariate statistical technique that uses food intake data to identify common subjacent dietary factors or patterns (Hu, 2002; Moeller et al., 2007). Cluster analysis, another multivariate method, aggregates individuals into relatively homogeneous subgroups with similar dietary characteristics. These techniques allow the classification of individuals into distinct groups or in groups according to food intake frequency; classification of foods or food groups according to their percentage energy contribution or mean amount consumed in grams; establishment of nutrient intake patterns; and combination of dietary and biochemical measurements (Hu, 2002; Moeller et al., 2007).

The association between dietary pattern and the prevalence of obesity and/or cardiovascular diseases has indicated a positive correlation between certain dietary patterns and indicators of these diseases (Berg et al., 2009; Howarth et al., 2007; Ma et al., 2003; Meyer et al., 2011; Newby et al., 2003; Neumann et al., 2007; Sherafat-kazemzadeh et al., 2010; Sichieri, 2002). Nevertheless, reviews on dietary patterns and their relationship with certain diseases have found data inconsistencies, signaling the need of more thorough studies on this theme (Bhupathiraju; Tucker, 2011; Kant, 2004; Togo et al., 2001).

Based on the high frequency of food intake underreporting among the obese, some food groups and/or nutrients in the dietary patterns of obese women classified as energy intake underreporters may vary, so more studies are needed to identify the intake particularities of this population. In our group, Ravelli (2013) found that women often underreported their energy intake and that underreporting was associated with a healthier dietary pattern than the pattern of women who reported their intake correctly. This suggests that underreporting involves foods that obese individuals should restrict.

5. Dietary approach of preoperative patients

The objective of bariatric surgery is to reduce energy intake and consequently promote weight loss, better quality of life, and the improvement of associated comorbidities. Long-term weight loss maintenance depends on the development of a multidisciplinary education program focusing on the surgery, making patients and family members aware of its risks and benefits, the importance of adhering to the dietary recommendations because of the anatomical and hormonal changes, and the resultant biopsychosocial and physical activity changes.

Once the type of surgery is selected, patients should undergo a nutritional assessment as soon as possible to identify possible nutritional deficiencies, establish a plan to promote dietary adequacy, and make sure they understand the dietary changes they will experience to prevent postoperative complications. Factors such as the patient's readiness for change, realistic expectations, general food and nutrition knowledge, and financial aspects must be investigated and clarified during the preoperative nutritional treatment.

5.1. Initial interventions and strategies for preoperative weight loss

Planning the nutritional intervention requires defining treatment objectives. Goals are individual and based on associated diseases, personal preferences, and habits mentioned in the nutritional anamnesis. Weight loss maintenance demands the adoption of proper food choice-related habits and practices, eating behaviors, and energy expenditure.

The preoperative nutritional approach may be collective or individual. We conduct a complete nutritional anamnesis in our first meeting with the patients and seize the opportunity to help them to improve their dietary habits, bond with them, destroy misconceptions and myths, and inform them about the surgery and the necessary postoperative dietary changes required by the surgery of choice.

5.1.1. Nutritional anamnesis

Nutritional anamnesis has a critical role in nutrition and health research. Its objective is to characterize the general nutritional status of an individual to determine the appropriate intervention.

Anamnesis consists of:

- Anthropometric assessment: preoperative weight, height, body mass index (BMI=kg/m^2), percentage of excess weight (%), and body composition determined by bioelectrical impedance analysis;
- History of weight and previous treatments: patients are asked about the details of their obesity history, unsuccessful weight loss treatments, life events that may have promoted weight changes, weight loss expectations, and previous clinical treatments;
- Biochemical parameters: includes the tests routinely requested by the surgeon and endocrinologist during the preoperative period as recommended by the Brazilian Society of Bariatric and Metabolic Surgery and American Society for Metabolic & Bariatric Surgery;
- Clinical history: assesses the patients' comorbidities and the drugs and supplements they are taking and verifies the presence of orthodontic and sight problems and of food allergies. Bowel movements, voiding habits, and menstrual frequency are also investigated;
- Smoking: the patients are asked about their smoking habits, including the number of cigarettes consumed per day;

- Alcohol intake: the patients are asked about their drinking habits, including amount and frequency;
- Food-related emotional aspect: the patients are asked about how their emotions affect their eating habits;
- Physical activity: the patients are asked about their physical endurance, the types of activity they performed in the past, and what they expect to achieve physically after surgery. At this time the patients are informed about the importance of starting a physical activity program supervised by a certified professional as soon as the surgeon releases them;
- Dietary history: collects information on snacking habits, mastication, fluid intake during meals, and daily water intake;
- Food preferences: investigates patients' food and preparation preferences, aversions, and intolerances;
- Food intake: the patients are asked about their habitual food intake during weekdays and weekend days; intake frequency of the main foods of each food group; meal number and location; food preferences and aversions; possible religious and/or cultural food restrictions; and food preparation techniques and purchasing habits to identify preparation problems or facilities. We also routinely ask the patients to make a food diary on three nonconsecutive days, including a weekend day, to better determine their food intake profiles.

We also take into account the reality of the patients, their jobs, routines, schedules, financial resources, literacy levels, and regional habits to personalize the intervention, otherwise it would be difficult to obtain good adherence to treatment.

The patients receive nutrition education based on the information collected by the nutritional anamneses, with emphasis on healthy food choices, the importance of consuming foods from all food groups, and the relationship between hunger and satiety. A personalized eating plan with lower energy content is created for the patients for them to start losing weight before surgery, reducing surgery risks and allowing us to assess their discipline.

The number and frequency of visits may vary according to the particularities of the patient and determination of the bariatric surgery team. The objective of the follow-ups is to assess adherence to the recommendations, weight loss, and changes in dietary habits, and to clarify surgery-related doubts. In the last visit prior to surgery, the patient and his/her companion receive verbal and written advice about the pre-and postoperative fluid diet.

Many issues are discussed with the patients in more detail during the visits, such as their need to lose 5% to 10% of their body weight before surgery, the preoperative eating plan, mastication, surgical techniques and resulting nutritional changes, healthy food choices, and specifics about the fluid diet that should be followed before and after surgery, always emphasizing healthy food choices and habits. The nutritional intervention also has the following cognitive objectives:

- The surgery helps the patient to limit food intake by reducing gastric volume and absorption area, depending on surgical technique, thereby promoting weight loss;

- The importance of the patient assuming a compromise with his/her health, since postoperative eating discipline is critical to avoid nutritional inadequacies and/or weight regain;
- The intake of energy-dense fluids and alcoholic beverages and early or excessive inclusion of simple sugars and fats may cause treatment failure or dumping syndrome;
- Dumping syndrome – definition, symptoms, how to avoid;
- Mastication – the patient must eat slowly to avoid the sensation of having food stuck on the way down, malaise, or even vomiting. This is valid for fluid and solid preparations;
- Advice and required dietary changes for the preoperative (fluid) and postoperative (fluid, soft, and general) periods, and foods that should be avoided after the surgery.

The advice regarding patients' new eating behavior should be provided by a dietician together with a psychologist to encourage patients to identify inappropriate eating behaviors and teach them new eating habits even before surgery. These recommendations increase postoperative adherence to the nutritional therapy and reduce the incidence of postoperative complications.

6. Dietary approach of postoperative patients

Nutritional counseling after surgery is essential because of all the changes patients must make to their eating habits. Follow-ups must be periodical to assess weight loss, encourage the adoption of healthy eating habits, clarify doubts, and identify possible nutritional inadequacies. Counseling is critical to ensure surgery success and avoid future complications.

Nutritional recommendations may vary by type of surgery, but all of them have similar diet therapy objectives: to reduce the work of the stomach and intestinal overload in the immediate postoperative period and to promote healthy food choices and habits using a diet plan associated with specific, personalized nutritional supplementation to meet the nutritional requirements of the patient.

Patient noncompliance with postoperative control programs is usually high, especially one year after surgery, which means lower adherence to the recommended healthy behaviors, and consequently, risk of bariatric surgery failure. Therefore, it is essential for the patient to learn and recognize the importance of adherence to treatment before the surgery.

6.1. Dietary changes

Ingestion is forbidden in the 24 hours that follow surgery, regardless of type. After this period the patient may start ingesting fluids. The objective of the fluid diet is to allow gastric rest and adaptation to small volumes, promote systemic hydration, ease the digestive process and gastric emptying, and prevent the ingestion of residues (Aills et al., 2008).

Our patients are placed on a fluid diet three days before surgery and recommended to stay on the diet until the twentieth day after surgery. This diet must consist exclusively of fluids. Patients receive verbal advice and a written document containing instructions regarding volume, fractioning, the foods they may and may not consume, a menu example, recipes, and supplementation. The preoperative fluid diet differs from the postoperative fluid diet only in volume. During the hospitalization period, which varies from two to four days, the patients are given a residue-free fluid diet consisting only of water, light-colored tea, sugar-free gelatin dessert, isotonic drinks, coconut water, and stock.

All diets are adapted to the type of surgery and the particularities of each patient. When our patients return for a follow-up visit fifteen days after the surgery, we verify the volume they are ingesting, meal fractioning, the use of protein and micronutrient supplements, daily water intake, voiding habits, bowel movements, possible eating difficulties, and physical signs of nutritional deficiencies. Our patients also receive verbal and written advice about the soft diet that should be started twenty days after the surgery.

The second follow-up visit occurs 25 to 35 days after surgery. During this visit, we advise patients about the general diet, examine them for physical signs of nutritional deficiencies, and collect information about food intake during the soft-diet period, such as amounts consumed, number of meals consumed per day, ingestion of the recommended nutrient supplements, water intake, voiding habits, bowel movements, and eating difficulties. We also advise the patients to start the general diet slowly, according to their recovery and food acceptance. The general diet (solid) should begin 35 days after surgery.

Bariatric surgery patients should be nutritionally monitored. Visiting the dietician regularly is extremely important because the small volume of the stomach greatly restricts nutrient intake. In the first months after surgery, nausea and vomiting are common; nevertheless, they must be investigated and the patients, counseled (Mechanick et al. 2009). The follow-up schedule may vary according to individual needs and possible surgery complications. Some patients even require special follow-up (Mechanick et al., 2009). We ask our patients to visit us once a month for five months after they start the general diet, then quarterly for six months, then semiannually or as needed.

Nutritional care after bariatric surgery has two objectives: the first is to adjust the energy and nutrient intakes necessary for tissue repair after surgery and for preserving lean body mass during extreme weight loss, and the second is to minimize the symptoms caused by surgery-induced changes, such as reflux, early satiety, and dumping syndrome (Aills et al., 2008).

The manner in which postoperative weight loss factors interact determines how surgery affects body weight in the short and long terms, hence the importance of knowing the weight loss pattern and related factors. Long-term follow-up is also advised to monitor the outcome and make sure that the surgery-related benefits are long-lived.

7. Dietary approaches to prevent and treat postoperative complications

The main comorbidities associated with obesity, such as diabetes and high blood pressure, improve significantly shortly after bariatric surgery, but other complications may arise given the surgery-induced anatomic and physiological changes. The most common postoperative

http://dx.doi.org/10.5772/58636

complications include nutritional deficiencies, anemia, dumping syndrome, vomiting, and alopecia.

Nutritional deficiencies (iron and anemia, calcium, vitamins D, B_{12}, B_6, and B_1, zinc, and protein-energy malnutrition) and their consequences may occur after surgery, especially in the long-term. The severity of these complications depends on the extension of the anatomic and physiological changes made to the gastrointestinal tract, as mentioned earlier. Nutritional deficiencies may cause severe morbidity and irreversible damage, and conventional supplementation is often not enough. Specific inadequacies must be corrected to restore normal serum levels and avoid greater consequences. It is essential to perform periodical tests as recommended by the guidelines to measure the serum levels of certain nutrients (Heber et al., 2010).

Patients who undergo mixed surgeries (RYGB) and mostly malabsorptive mixed surgeries (BPD) require specific monitoring and supplementation, especially in the first year after surgery. Additional supplements of iron and calcium, water-soluble vitamins, and vitamins A and D are prescribed more often to BPD-DS (55%) patients than to RYGB (26%) patients (Aasheim et al., 2009).

Bariatric patients require a minimum daily mineral and vitamin supplementation of one (AGB) to two (RYGB, BPD, and SG) multivitamin and multimineral tablets, 1200-1500 mg of elemental calcium in the form of citrate divided throughout the day, 3000 IU of vitamin D (to keep serum 25(OH)D above 30ng/mL), and enough vitamin B_{12} to maintain normal serum values. Vitamin B_{12} can be taken orally, sublingually, intranasally, or intramuscularly as follows: 350 mcg orally per day; or 500 mcg intranasally per week; or 1000 mcg intramuscularly per month; or 3000 mcg intramuscularly semiannually. Finally, the amount of folic acid present in multivitamins is adequate (400 mcg) (Mechanick et al., 2009; Mechanick, et al., 2013).

The vitamin B_{12} status of all patients undergoing bariatric surgery, regardless of type, should be assessed before surgery, and of patients who lost the lower part of their stomach (SG, RYGB and BPD), should also be assessed annually after surgery. Supplementation with 1000 ug or more of crystalline vitamin B_{12} daily may be necessary to maintain adequate serum levels of this vitamin (Kehagias et al., 2011).

Conventional or additional supplementation should provide 45 to 60 mg of iron per day. Iron serum levels should be monitored in all bariatric surgery patients and individuals with iron-deficiency anemia. Anemia treatment includes the prescription of 150 to 200 mg of elemental iron orally per day in the form of iron sulfate, fumarate, or gluconate. Vitamin C may be taken simultaneously to increase iron absorption. Intravenous iron infusion is indicated for patients with severe deficiency, oral intolerance, or refractory anemia due to severe iron malabsorption. Nutritional anemia stemming from malabsorptive bariatric surgeries also include deficiency of vitamin B_{12}, folic acid, protein-energy, copper, selenium, and zinc, so these deficiencies must be assessed and corrected in patients with persistent anemia (Aills et al., 2008).

Protein-energy malnutrition is usually accompanied by hypoalbuminemia, alopecia, asthenia, and anemia. Some studies have found that two years after surgery, 5% to 13% of RYGB patients and 3% to 18% of BPD patients have hypoalbuminemia. Bariatric patients should ingest at least

60 grams of protein a day, or 1.5g/kg of the ideal body weight a day, or if necessary 2.1g/kg of the ideal body weight a day (Mechanick, et al., 2013).

Bone loss may occur in the long run, especially in women, so complete assessment of calcium metabolism is essential to make sure that the ingested and absorbed amounts are enough to prevent metabolic bone disease. RYGB, BPD, or BPD-DS patients must take calcium citrate and vitamin D [ergocalciferol (D_2) or cholecalciferol (D_3)] orally to prevent or minimize secondary hyperparathyroidism without inducing hypercalciuria. In severe cases of vitamin D malabsorption, oral doses may be increased to 50,000 IU one to three times a week or even daily. Hypophosphatemia is usually due to vitamin D deficiency. An oral phosphate supplement should be taken when the serum level is in the 1.5 to 2.5 mg/dL bracket (Mechanick, et al., 2013).

Vitamin A deficiency may cause vision problems. Supplementation, isolated or combined with other fat-soluble vitamins, is recommended for patients who undergo purely malabsorptive procedures, such as BPD or BPD-DS. There is no evidence to suggest that bariatric surgery patients should be routinely screened for low levels of essential fatty acids, vitamin E, or vitamin K. However, health care providers should consider vitamin K assessment when they find an established deficiency of fat-soluble vitamins (hepatopathy, coagulopathy, or osteoporosis) (Aasheim et al., 2009).

There is also no evidence to suggest that routine selenium screening or supplementation is necessary after bariatric surgery. Nevertheless, health care providers should measure the serum selenium levels of patients who undergo malabsorptive surgeries or of patients with anemia, fatigue, persistent diarrhea, cardiomyopathy, or metabolic bone disease. Zinc deficiency should be assessed routinely in BPD or BPD-DS patients or patients with alopecia, ageusia, and dysgeusia (Aills et al., 2008).

Copper supplementation (2 mg/day) should be included as part of the supplementation routine. Consider measuring the serum copper level of patients with persistent anemia, neutropenia, myeloneuropathy, and poor wound healing. Patients being treated for zinc deficiency and alopecia should take 1 mg of copper for each 8 to 15 mg of zinc since zinc supplementation may cause copper deficiency (Mechanick, et al., 2013).

Vomiting may occur in the postoperative period, especially in the first months after surgery, and is generally precipitated by eating more than the stomach can hold or not chewing well. It may also indicate other problems, such as stenosis or intolerance to solid foods (Fujioka, 2005).

Intolerance to solid foods is the main characteristic of patients who are not chewing foods well enough, especially foods that are harder to chew, such as meats, non-starchy vegetables, and all foods with a more fibrous consistency. These patients prefer softer foods, such as soups (with a high proportion of carbohydrates), pasta, puree, soufflé, ice cream, cookies, certain savory snacks and pastries, and other foods that do not require much effort to chew and swallow.

After surgery bariatric patients may also experience trauma or fear for not knowing how much food to put in their mouths at a time or how much to chew before swallowing, and end up feeling nauseated, vomiting, or feeling that the bolus got stuck somewhere between the throat and the stomach.

Patients with persistent vomiting who chew well but are intolerant to solids should be specifically examined for stenosis by the surgeon to rule out functional disorders, even if the intolerance developed postoperatively (Fujioka, 2005).

Frequent vomiting may cause thiamine deficiency. Thiamine should be part of the conventional supplementation, as the other water-soluble vitamins. Susceptible patients include those with rapid weight loss, prolonged vomiting, excessive alcohol intake, neuropathy, encephalopathy, and heart failure. Patients with suspected or established severe thiamine deficiency should receive 500mg of intravenous thiamine daily for three to five days, followed by 250 mg daily for three to five days until the symptoms subside. Health care providers should consider further supplementation with 100mg orally per day for an indeterminate period or until the risk factors are eliminated (Mechanick, et al., 2009).

Dumping syndrome is a common bariatric surgery complication experienced by roughly 70% of RYGB patients. Foods with high osmolarity, such as those with high sugar content, cause osmotic overload in the small intestine (Fujioka, 2005; Mechanick et al., 2009). The symptoms include hypoglycemia, abdominal pain, nausea, diarrhea, rubor, and tachycardia (Elliot, 2003; Merchanick et al., 2009). Late dumping syndrome symptoms may be caused by reactive hypoglycemia, normally controlled through diet or treated prophylactically with half a cup of orange juice roughly one hour after a meal (Mechanick et al., 2009).

Bariatric patients must learn about dumping syndrome, its symptoms, and which foods to avoid before surgery. During the nutrition education process, we strongly encourage our patients to restrict the intake of simple sugars and reduce the intake of high-fat foods before and after surgery. Patients are also encouraged to eat small amounts at a time, avoid ingesting fluids thirty minutes before and after a solid meal, prefer complex carbohydrates to simple ones, and increase protein intake.

Alopecia, classified as a nutritional complication of bariatric surgery, occurs mainly in the first year after surgery, a time of intense weight loss and patients' adaptation to diet and their new gastrointestinal system. Nutritional deficiency-related alopecia is mainly associated with the deficiency of zinc, iron, proteins, and essential fatty acids, so requires proper supplementation.

Most bariatric patients may experience one or more nutritional deficiencies, justifying the need of lifelong vitamin and mineral supplementation after surgery, and macronutrient supplementation when necessary. Thus, the dietician assumes the critical role of preventing and correcting nutritional changes after bariatric surgery.

8. Dietary approach for preventing weight regain

Bariatric surgery promotes the control of obesity, not the cure, and complications may occur at any time (Novais et al., 2010). Weight loss after bariatric surgery is clearly visible, with consequent improvement of the comorbidities and quality of life. Therefore, weight loss is considered one of the main parameters for defining bariatric surgery success (Brolin, 2002; Brolin, 2007; Silver et al., 2006; Novais et al., 2010). Researchers unanimously agree that a successful outcome requires an excess weight loss (%EWL) of at least 50% and the long-term maintenance of the weight loss (Capella, Capella, 1996; Brolin et al., 1994; Brolin, 2002; Fobi, 2004; Brolin 2007; Silver et al., 2006; Novais, 2010).

Weight regain after surgery may be promoted by physiological adaptations of the gastrointestinal tract. Adoption of a healthy lifestyle protects bariatric patients from old habits directly related to obesity. This new behavior is important to maintain the new body weight in the long run, so the support of a certified multidisciplinary team is critical (Bond et al., 2004; Novais et al., 2010).

Weight loss and control after surgery are checked routinely. Many indicators are used for this purpose, such as BMI, percentage of the initial weight loss, and percentage of excess weight loss. We use the latter in our practice.

Most of the weight loss occurs in the six months after surgery, when food intake restriction is greater (Novais et al., 2010). Patients submitted to malabsorptive procedures may lose 0.2 – 0.5 kg per day, achieving a loss of 18 – 40.5 kg in the first three months after surgery. The weight lost peaks between 12 and 18 months after surgery (Mechanick et al., 2009, Novais et al., 2010).

Small weight loss after surgery should be investigated by the multidisciplinary team. The dietician must check the patient's food habits, especially the intake of energy-dense foods. Some studies found that even bariatric patients may regain weight (Kaplan, 2005; Livingston, 2005), especially three to five years after surgery (Brolin *et al.*, 1994; Buchwald et al., 2004; Mechanick et al., 2009). Obesity may recur because it is a chronic disease. Patients must understand that weight fluctuations are normal and perfectly acceptable. Weight-loss plateau or even a small weight regain are part of the normal weight loss process. Professionals must emphasize on the better quality of life, healthy behaviors, and better health status instead of percentage of excess weight loss as a measure of success.

Our group (Novais, 2009) investigated the food intake, weight history, and quality of life of 141 females two years after bariatric surgery and found that 84.4% lost more than 50% of their excess perioperative weight. Significant weight loss occurred in the first six months after surgery and stabilized two years after surgery. About 15% of the patients regained part of their excess weight. In another study our group (Fogaça, 2009) assessed the factors associated with weight regain in women two years after bariatric surgery and found that the resting energy expenditure adjusted for total and lean body mass, and the serum lipids, glucose, insulin, and leptin of women who regained more than 10% of their weight did not differ significantly from those of the controls-women who did not regain weight.

Food habits impact weight loss speed and long-term maintenance. Hence, dieticians and psychologists work side by side with bariatric patients with eating disorders that may promote weight regain. Psychologists help patients to find skills that satisfy their emotional needs and dieticians help them to effectively learn to nourish their minds and bodies, enabling them to deal with their emotions, desires, and biological needs.

The relationship between psychologist and dietician is essential to treat each patient individually. Many patients do not assimilate so many changes, justifying their weight regain or replacement of a symptom by another eating disorder or compulsive behavior. Others manage to carry out the necessary changes, improving their emotional status and reducing their levels of anxiety and depression. The importance of psychological and sometimes psychiatric follow-up is clear as it helps to improve patients' quality of life and interpersonal relationships.

Weight regain after bariatric surgery is a reality, hence the need of prospective studies with patients in line for bariatric surgery and the critical work of a multidisciplinary team to provide the best treatment possible and ensure a successful outcome, not only in terms of weight loss but also in terms of body nourishment and quality of life.

9. Final considerations

As a result of the knowledge we have accumulated in our clinical and research practice and consonant with the literature, we can state that bariatric surgery changes the nourishment process substantially, implying the need of permanently monitoring the patients' nutritional status. This practice should begin already in the waiting line for bariatric surgery because nutritional deficiencies may occur in obese individuals despite their excessive food intake; they may either have a poor diet.

In addition to anthropometric assessment, patients should undergo a thorough assessment of the signs and symptoms associated with nutritional deficiencies, measurement of serum nutrient levels, and food intake assessment. Food intake assessment has technical and operational limitations, but it is an essential tool for dietary diagnosis and prescription, and for food and nutrition education. Food and nutrition education must be based on science and supported by the other professionals in the team. In addition to a dietician, a psychologist is needed to help patients to develop the skills they need to practice self-care. Furthermore, although surgery improves the metabolic disorders associated with adipose tissue, nutritional deficiencies should always be a target of concern, prophylactic intervention, and monitoring. Therefore, a multidisciplinary health care team is critically needed for providing the lifelong care required by bariatric patients.

Author details

Patrícia Fátima Sousa Novais[1,2,3], Flávia Andreia Marin[1,2,3], Alex Harley Crisp[1,2,3], Irineu Rasera Junior[1,2,3], Celso Vieira de Souza Leite[1] and Maria Rita Marques de Oliveira[1,2,3]

1 Universidade Estadual Paulista, Botucatu SP, Brazil

2 Universidade Estadual Paulista, Araraquara SP, Brazil

3 Clinica Bariátrica – Hospital dos Fornecedores de Cana, Piracicaba SP, Brazil

References

[1] Aasheim, ET., Hofsø, D., Hjelmesaeth, J., Birkeland, KI., Bøhmer, T. (2008). Vitamin status in morbidly obese patients: a cross-sectional study. *American Journal of Clinical Nutrition*, Vol. 87, No. 2, pp. 362-369, ISSN 0002-9165.

[2] Aasheim, ET., Björkman, S., Søvik, TT., Engström, M., Hanvold, SE., Mala, T., Olbers, T., Bøhmer T. (2009). Vitamin status after bariatric surgery: a randomized study of gastric bypass and duodenal switch. *American Journal of Clinical Nutrition*, Vol. 90, No. 1, pp. 15-22, ISSN 0002-9165.

[3] Abbot, JM., Thomson, CA., Ranger-Moore, J., Teixeira, PJ., Lohman, TG., Taren, DL., Cussler, E., Going, SB., Houtkooper, LB. (2008). Psychosocial and behavioral profile and predictors of self-reported energy inderreporting in obese middle-aged women. Journal of the American Dietetic Association, Vol. 108, No. 1, pp. 114-119, ISSN 0002-8223.

[4] Aills, L., Blankenship, J., Buffington, C., Furtado, M., Parrott, J. (2008). ASMBS Allied Health Nutritional Guidelines for the Surgical Weight Loss Patient. *Surgery for Obesity and Related Diseases*, Vol. 4, pp. 73-108, ISSN 1550-7289.

[5] Anjos, LA., Souza, DR., Rossato, SL. (2009). Desafios na medição quantitativa da ingestão alimentar em estudos populacionais. *Revista de Nutrição*, Vol. 22, No. 1, pp. 151-161, ISSN 1415-5273.

[6] Berg, C., Lappas, G., Wolk, A., Strandhagen, E., Torén, K., Rosengren, A., Thelle, D., Lissner, L. (2009). Eating patterns and portion size associated with obesity in Swedish population. Appetite, Vol. 52, No. 1, pp. 21-26, ISSN 0195-6663.

[7] Bekri, S., Gual, P., Anty, R., Luciani, N., Dahman, M., Ramesh, B., et al. (2006). Increased adipose tissue expression of hepcidin in severe obesity is independent from diabetes and NASH. *Gastroenterology*, Vol. 131, pp.788-96, ISSN 0016-5085.

[8] Bhupathiraju, SN., Tucker, KL. (2011). Coronary heart disease prevention: nutrients, foods, and dietary patterns. *Clinica Chimica Acta*, Vol. 412, No. 17-18, pp. 1493-1514, ISSN 0009-8981. 2011, 412:1493–1514.

[9] Black, AE., Goldberg, GR., Jebb, SA., Livingstone, MB., Cole TJ., Prentice AM. (1991). Critical evaluation of energy intake data using fundamental principles of energy physiology: 2. Evaluating the results of published surveys. *European Journal of Clinical Nutrition*, Vol. 45, No. 12, pp. 583-599, ISSN 0954-3007.

[10] Black, AE. (2000) Critical evaluation of energy intake using the Goldberg cut-off for energy intake: basal metabolic rate. A practical guide to its calculation, use and limitations. *International Journal of Obesity and Related Metabolic Disorders*, Vol. 24, No. 9, pp. 1119-1130, ISSN 0307-0565.

[11] Black, AE., Cole, TJ. (2001). Biased over-or under-reporting is characteristic of individuals whether over time or by different assessment methods. Journal of the American Dietetic Association, Vol. 101, No. 1, pp. 70-80, ISSN 0002-8223.

[12] Bloomberg, RD., Fleishman, A., Nalle, JE., Herron, DM., Kini, S. (2005). Nutritional deficiencies following bariatric surgery: what have we learned? *Obesity Surgery,* Vol. 15, pp. 145-154, ISSN 0960-8923.

[13] Bond, DS., Evans, RK., Demaria, EJ., Meador, RN., Warren, BJ., Shannon, KA., et al. (2004). A conceptual application of health behavior theory in the design and implementation of a successful surgical weight loss program. *Obesity Surgery,* Vol. 14, pp. 849-56, ISSN 0960-8923.

[14] Brolin, RL., Robertson, LB., Kenler, HA., Cody, RP. Weight loss and dietary intake after vertical banded gastroplasty and Roux-en-Y gastric bypass. (1994). *Annals of Surgery*, Vol. 220, No. 6, pp 782-790, ISSN 0003-4932.

[15] Brolin, RE. (2002). Bariatric surgery and long-term control of morbid obesity. *JAMA,* Vol. 288, pp. 2793-2796, ISSN 0098-7484.

[16] Brolin, RE., LaMarca, LB., Kenler, HA., Cody, RP. (2002). Malabsorptive gastric bypass in patients with superobesity. *Journal of Gastrointestinal Surgery,* Vol. 6, pp. 195–203, ISSN 1091-255X.

[17] Brolin, RE. (2007). Weight gain after short-and long-limb gastric bypass in patients followed for longer than 10 years. *Annals of Surgery*, Vol. 246, No 1, pp. 163-164, ISSN 0003-4932.

[18] Brouwer, DA., van Beek, J., Ferwerda, H., Brugman, AM., van der Klis, FR., van der Heiden, HJ., Muskiet, FA. (1998). Rat adipose tissue rapidly accumulates and slowly releases an orally-administered high vitamin D dose. British Journal of Nutrition, Vol. 79, No. 6, pp. 527-532, ISSN 0007-1145.

[19] Buchwald, H., Avidor, Y., Braunwald, E., Jensen, MD., Pories, W., Fahrbach, K., Schoelles. (2004). Bariatric surgery: a systematic review and meta-analysis. *JAMA,* Vol. 292, No. 14, pp. 1724-1737, ISSN 0098-7484.

[20] Censani, M., Stein, EM., Shane, E., Oberfield, SE., McMahon, DJ., Lerner, S., Fennoy, I. (2013). Vitamin D Deficiency Is Prevalent in Morbidly Obese Adolescents Prior to Bariatric Surgery. *ISRN Obesity*, Vol. 2013, pp. 284516, ISSN 2090-9496.

[21] Capella, JF., Capella, RF. (1996). The weight reduction operation of choice: vertical banded gastroplasty or gastric bypass? *The American Journal of Surgery,* Vol. 171, pp. 74-79, ISSN 0002-9610.

[22] Chen, SB., Lee, YC., Ser, KH., Chen, JC., Chen, SC., Hsieh, HF., et al. (2009). Serum C-reactive protein and white blood cell count in morbidly obese surgical patients. *Obesity Surgery,* Vol. 19, No. 2, pp. 461-466, ISSN 0960-8923.

[23] Carlin, AM., Rao, DS., Meslemani, AM., Genaw, JA., Parikh, NJ., Levy, S., Bhan, A., Talpos, GB. (2006). Prevalence of vitamin D depletion among morbidly obese patients seeking gastric surgery. *Surgery for Obsesity and Related Diseases*, Vol. 2, No. 2, pp. 98-103, ISSN 1550-7289.

[24] Casagrande, DS., Repetto, G., Mottin, CC., Schneider, R., Rizzolli, J., Moretto, M., Padoin, AV., Schaan, BD. (2010). Bone mineral density and nutritional profile in morbidly obese women. *Obesity Surgery*, Vol. 20, No. 10, pp. 1372-1379, ISSN 0960-8923.

[25] Cimbek, A., Gürsoy, G., Kirnap, NG., Acar, Y., Kiliç, Z., Güngör, F., Ozasik, I. (2012). Relation of obesity with serum 25 hydroxy vitamin D3 levels in type 2 diabetic patients. *Journal of Research in Medical Sciences*, Vol. 17, No. 12, pp. 1119-1123, ISSN 1735-1995.

[26] Ducloux, R., Nobécourt, E., Chevallier, JM., Ducloux, H., Elian, N., Altman, JJ. (2011). Vitamin D deficiency before bariatric surgery: should supplement intake be routinely prescribed?. *Obesity Surgery*, Vol. 21, No. 5, pp. 556-560, ISSN 0960-8923.

[27] de Luis, DA., Pacheco, D., Izaola, O., Terroba, MC., Cuellar, L., Cabezas, G. (2013). Micronutrient status in morbidly obese women before bariatric surgery. *Surgery for obesity and related diseases*, Vol. 9, No. 2, pp. 323-327, ISSN 1550-7289.

[28] Dodell, GB., Albu, JB., Attia, L., McGinty, J., Pi-Sunyer, FX., Laferrère, B. (2012). The bariatric surgery patient: lost to follow-up; from morbid obesity to severe malnutrition. *Endocrine Practice*, Vol. 18, No. 2, pp. 21-25, ISSN 1530-891X.

[29] Dodd, KW., Guenther, PM., Freedman, LS., Subar, AF., Kipnis, V., Midthune, D., Tooze, JA., Krebs-Smith, SM. (2006). Statistical Methods for Estimating Usual Intake of Nutrients and Foods: A Review of Theory. *Journal of the American Dietetic Association*, Vol. 106, No. 10, pp. 1640-1650, ISSN 0002-8223.

[30] Duran de Campos, C., Dalcanale, L., Pajecki, D., Garrido, AB Jr., Halpern, A. (2008). Calcium intake and metabolic bone disease after eight years of Roux-en-Y gastric bypass. *Obesity Surgery*, Vol. 18, No. 4, pp.386-390, ISSN 0960-8923.

[31] Drygalski, AV., Andris, DA., Nuttleman, PR., Jackson, S., Klein, J., Wallace, JR. (2011). Anemia after bariatric surgery cannot be explained by iron deficiency alone: results of a large cohort study. *Surgery* for *Obesity and Related Diseases*, Vol. 7, pp. 151-156, ISSN 1550-7289.

[32] Ernst, B., Thurnheer, M., Schmid, SM., Schultes, B. (2009). Evidence for the necessaty to systematically assess micronutrient status to bariatric surgery. *Obesity Surgery*, Vol. 19, No. 1, pp. 66-73, ISSN 0960-8923.

[33] Elliot, K. (2003). Nutritional considerations after bariatric surgery. *Critical Care Nurse*, Vol. 26, No. 2, pp. 133-138, ISSN 0887-9303.

[34] Fogaça, KCP. (2009). *Investigação de Fatores envolvidos na Recuperação de Peso após Derivação Gástrica.* 121 f. Tese (Doutorado em Alimentos e Nutrição) – Universidade Estadual Paulista "Julio de Mesquita Filho"/UNESP, Araraquara/SP.

[35] Fobi, MA. (2004). Surgical treatment of obesity: a review. *Journal of the National Medical Association,* Vol. 96, No. 1, pp. 61-75. ISSN 0027-9684.

[36] Fish, E., Beverstein, G., Olson, D., Reinhardt, S., Garren, M., Gould, J. (2010). Vitamin D status of morbidly obese bariatric surgery patients. *Journal of Surgical Research,* Vol. 164, No. 2, pp. 198-202, ISSN 0022-4804.

[37] Flancbaum, L., Belsley, S., Drake, V., Colarusso, T., Tayler, E. (2006). Preoperative nutritional status of patients undergoing Roux-en-Y gastric bypass for morbid obesity. *Journal of Gastrointestinal Surgery, Vol.* 10, No. 7, pp. 1033-1037, ISSN 1091-255X.

[38] Fujioka, K. (2005). Follow-up of nutritional and metabolic problems after bariatric surgery. *Diabetes Care,* Vol. 28, pp. 481 – 484, ISSN 0149-5992.

[39] Gasteyger, C., Suter, M., Gaillard, RC., Giusti, V. (2008). Nutritional deficiencies after Roux-en-Y gastric bypass for morbid obesity often cannot be prevented by standard multivitamin supplementation. *American Journal of Clinical Nutrition,* Vol. 87, n. 5, pp. 1128-1133, ISSN 1938-3207.

[40] Gibson, RS. Principles of nutritional assessment 2ed. New York: Oxford University Press, 2005.

[41] Goldberg, GR., Black, AE., Jebb, SA., Cole, TJ., Murgatroyd, PR., Coward, WA., Prentice, AM. (1991). Critical evaluation of energy intake data using fundamental principles of energy physiology: 1. Derivation of cut-off limits to identify under-recording. *European Journal of Clinical Nutrition,* Vol. 45, No. 12, pp. 569-581, ISSN 0954-3007.

[42] Howarth, NC., Huang, TT., Roberts, SB., Lin, BH., McCrory, MA. (2007). Eating patterns and dietary composition in relation BMI in younger and older adults. *International Journal of Obesity,* Vol. 31, No. 4, pp. 675-684, ISSN 0307-0565.

[43] Heber, D., Greenway, FL., Kaplan, LM., Livingston, E., Salvador, J., Still, C. (2010). Endocrine and Nutritional Management of the Post-Bariatric Surgery Patient: An Endocrine Society Clinical Practice Guideline. *The Journal of Clinical Endocrinology and Metabolism,* Vol. 95, No. 11, pp. 4823–4843, ISSN 0021-972X

[44] Hu, FB. (2002). Dietary pattern analysis: a new direction in nutritional epidemiology. *Current Opinion in Lipidology,* Vol. 13, No. 1, pp. 3-9, ISSN 0957-9672.

[45] Jastrzębska-Mierzyńska, M., Ostrowska, L., Hady, HR., Dadan, J. (2012). Assessment of dietary habits, nutritional status and blood biochemical parameters in patients prepared for bariatric surgery: a preliminary study. *Wideochir Inne Tech Malo Inwazyjne,* Vol. 7, No. 3, pp. 156-165, ISSN 1895-4588.

[46] Johnson, RK. (2002). Dietary intake – how do we measure what people are really eating?. *Obesity Research*, Vol. 12, No. 1, pp. 63S-68S, ISSN 1071-7323.

[47] Kaplan, LM. (2005). Gastrointestinal management of the bariatric surgery patient. *Gastroenterology Clinics of North America*. Vol. 34, No. 1, pp. 105-125, ISSN 0889-8553.

[48] Kant, AK. (2004). Dietary Patterns and Health Outcomes. *Journal of the Ameican Dietetic Association*, Vol. 104, No. 4, pp. 615-635, ISSN 0002-8223.

[49] Kehagias, I., Karamanakos, SN., Argentou, M., Kalfarentzos, F. (2011). Randomized clinical trial of laparoscopic Roux-en-Y gastric bypass versus laparoscopic sleeve gastrectomy for the management of patients with BMI <50 kg/m2. *Obesity Surgery*, Vol. 21, No. 11, pp. 1650-1656, ISSN 0960-8923.

[50] Kimmons, JE., Blanck, HM., Tohill, BC., Zhang, J., Khan, LK. (2006). Associations between body mass index and the prevalence of low micronutrient levels among US adults. *Medscape General Medicine*, Vol. 8, No. 4, pp. 59, ISSN 1531-0132.

[51] Kohli, R., Stefater, MA., Inge, TH. (2011). Molecular insights from bariatric surgery. *Reviews in Endocrine and Metabolism Disorders*, Vol. 12, No. 3, pp. 211-217. ISSN 1389-9155.

[52] Lichtman, SW., Pisarska, K., Berman, ER., Pestone, M., Dowling, H., Offenbacher, E., Weisel, H., Matthews, DE., Heymsfield, SB. Discrepancy between self-reported and actual caloric intake and exercise in obese subjects. *New England Journal of Medicine*, Vol. 327, No. 27, pp. 1893-1898, ISSN 0028-4793.

[53] Livingston, EH. (2005). Complications of bariatric surgery. *The Surgical clinics of North America*, Vol. 85, No. 4, pp. 853-868, ISSN 0039-6109.

[54] Macdiarmid, J., Blundell, J. (1998). Assessing dietary intake: who, what and why of under-reporting. *Nutrition Research Reviews*, Vol. 11, No. 2, pp. 231-253, ISSN 0954-4224.

[55] Ma, Y., Bertone, ER., Stanek, EJ., Reed, GW., Habert, JR., Cohen, NL., Merriam, PA., Ockene, IS. (2003). Association between Eating Patterns and obesity in free-living US Adult Population. *American Journal of Epidemiology*, Vol. 158, No. 1, pp. 85-92, ISSN 0002-9262.

[56] Meyer, J., Doring, A., Herder, C., Roden, M., Koenin, W., Thorand, B. (2011). Dietary patterns, subclinical inflammation, incident coronary heart disease and mortality in middle-aged men from the MONICA/KORA Augsburg cohort study. *European Journal of Clinical Nutrition*, Vol. 65, No. 7, pp. 800-807, ISSN 0954-3007.

[57] Mechanick, JI., Kushner, RF., Sugerman, HJ., Gonzalez-Campoy, JM., Collazo-Clavell, ML., Spitz, AF., et al. (2009). American Association of Clinical Endocrinologists, the Obesity Society, and American Society for Metabolic & Bariatric Surgery Medical Guidelines for Clinical Practice for the Perioperative Nutritional, Metabolic, and

Nonsurgical Support of the Bariatric Surgery Patient. *Obesity*, Vol. 17, Suppl 1, pp. 1-70. ISSN 1930-7381.

[58] Mechanick, JI., Youdim, A., Jones, DB., Garvey, WT., Hurley, DL., McMahon, MM., Heinberg, LJ., Kushner, R., Adams, TD., Shikora, S., Dixon, JB., Brethauer, S. (2013). Clinical Practice Guidelines for the Perioperative Nutritional, Metabolic, and Nonsurgical Support of the Bariatric Surgery Patient--2013 Update : Cosponsored by American Association of Clinical Endocrinologists, The Obesity Society, and American Society for Metabolic & Bariatric Surgery. *Surgery for Obesity and Related Disease*, Vol. 8, No. 2, pp. 159-191, ISSN 1550-7289.

[59] Menendéz, E. (2009). Subjects, knowledge, and structures: an introduction to relational focus in the study of collective health. São Paulo: HUCITEC.

[60] Miller, GD., Nicklas, BJ., Fernandez, A. Serial changes in inflammatory biomarkers after Roux-en-Y gastric bypass surgery. (2011). *Surgery for Obesity and Related Diseases*, Vol. 7, No. 5, pp. 618-624, ISSN 150-7289.

[61] Moizé, V., Deulofeu, R., Torres, F., Osaba, JM., Vidal. J. (2011). Nutritional intake and prevalence of nutritional deficiencies prior to surgery in a Spanish morbidly obese population. *Obesity Surgery*, Vol. 21, No. 9, pp. 1382-1288, ISSN 0960-8923.

[62] Neumann, AICP., Martins, IS., Marcopito, LF., Araujo, EAC. (2007). Padrões alimentares associados a fatores de risco para doenças cardiovasculares entre residentes de um município brasileiro. *Revista Panamericana de Salud Pública*, Vol. 22, No. 5, pp. 329–339, ISSN 1020-4989.

[63] Newby, PK., Muller, D., Hallfrisch, J., Qiao, N., Andre, R., Tucker, KL. (2003). Dietary patterns and changes in body mass index and waist circumference in adults. *American Journal of Clinical Nutrition*, Vol. 77, No. 6, pp. 1417-1425, ISSN 0002-9165.

[64] Nicoletti, CF., Lima, TP., Donadelli, SP., Salgado, WJr., Marchini, JS., Nonino, CB. (2013). New look at nutritional care for obese patient candidates for bariatric surgery. *Surgery for Obesity and Related Diseases*, Vol. 9, No. 4, pp. 520-525, ISSN 1550-7289.

[65] Novais, PSF. (2009). Avaliação dos resultados da cirurgia bariátrica sobre o peso corporal, o consumo alimentar e a qualidade de vida de indivíduos no pós-cirúrgico tardio. 122 f. Dissertação (Mestrado em Alimentos e Nutrição). Universidade Estadual Paulista "Julio de Mesquita Filho" /UNESP, Araraquara/SP.

[66] Novais, PF., Rasera Junior, I., Leite, CV., Oliveira, MR. (2010). Evolução e classificação do peso corporal em relação aos resultados da cirurgia bariátrica: derivação gástrica em Y de Roux. *Arquivos Brasileiros de Endocrinologia e Metabologia*, Vol. 54, No. 3, pp. 303-310, ISSN 0004-2730.

[67] Novais, PF., Rasera, IJr., Leite, CV., Marin, FA., de Oliveira, MR. (2012). Food intake in women two years or more after bariatric surgery meets adequate intake requirements. *Nutrition Research*, Vol. 32, No. 5, pp. 335-341, ISSN 0271-5317.

[68] Pories, WJ. (2008). Bariatric surgery: risks and rewards. *Journal of Clinical Endocrinology and Metabolism,* Vol 93, pp. S89–S96, ISNN 0021-972X.

[69] Quesada, KR. Subnotificação da ingestão energética entre obesas candidatas a cirurgia bariátrica. Araraquara, SP, Brazil, 2011. Dissertation (master's degree) – Faculty of Pharmaceutical Sciences, UNESP. Graduate Program in Food and Nutrition.

[70] Ravelli, MN. Padrão alimentar de mulheres obesas que subnotificam ou não a ingestão energética. Araraquara, SP, Brazil, 2013. Dissertation (master's degree) – Faculty of Pharmaceutical Sciences, UNESP. Graduate Program in Food and Nutrition.

[71] Rennie, KL., Coward, A., Jebb, SA. (2007). Estimating under-reporting of energy intake in dietary surveys using an individualized method. British Journal of Nutrition, Vol. 97, No. 6, pp. 1169-1176, ISSN 0007-1145.

[72] Rodieux, F., Giusti, V., D' Alessio, DA., Suter, M., Tappy L. (2008). Effects of gastric bypass and gastric banding on glucose kinetics and gut hormone release. *Obesity (Silver Spring), Vol.* 16, pp. 2298-2305, ISSN 1930-7381.

[73] Ruz, M., Carrasco, F., Rojas, P., Codoceo, J., Inostroza, J., Rebolledo, A., et al. (2009). Iron absorption and iron status are reduced after Roux-en-Y gastric bypass. *American Journal of Clinical Nutrition,* Vol. 90, pp. 527–532, ISSN 0002-9165.

[74] Sherafat-Kazemzadeh, R., Egtesadi, S., Mirmiran, P., Gohari, M,, Farahani, SJ., Esfahani, FH., Vafa, MR;, Hedayati, M., Azizi, F. (2010). Dietary patterns by reduced rank regression predicting changes in obesity indices in a cohort study: Tehran Lipid and Glucose Study. *Asia Pacific Journal of Clinical Nutrition,* Vol. 19, No. 1, pp. 22-32, ISSN 0964-7058.

[75] Sichieri, R. (2002). Dietary Patterns and Their Associations with Obesity in the Brazilian City of Rio de Janeiro. *Obesity Research,* Vol. 10, No. 1, pp. 42-48, ISSN 1071-7323.

[76] Saltzman, E., Karl, JP. (2013). Nutrient deficiencies after gastric bypass surgery. *Annual Review of Nutrition,* Vol. 33, pp. 183-203, ISSN 0199-9885.

[77] Scagliusi, FB., Ferriolli, E., Pfrimer, K., Laureano, C., Cunha, CS., Gualano, B., Lourenço, BH., Lancha, AHJr. (2009). Characteristics of women who frequently underreport their energy intake: a doubly labelled water study. *European Journal of Clinical Nutrition,* Vol. 63, No. 10, pp. 1192-1199, ISSN 0954-3007.

[78] Schweiger, C., Weiss, R., Berry, E., Keidar, A. (2010). Nutritional deficiencies in bariatric surgery candidates. *Obesity Surgery,* Vol. 20, No. 2, pp.193-197, ISSN 0960-8923.

[79] Schoeller, DA. (1999). Recent advances from application of doubly labeled water to measurement of human energy expenditure. Journal of Nutrition, Vol. 129, No. 10, pp. 1765-1768, ISSN 0022-3166.

[80] Signori, C., Zalesin, KC., Franklin, B., Miller, WL., Mac-Cullough, PA. (2010). Effect of Gastric Bypass on Vitamin D and Secondary Hyperparathyroidism. *Obesity Surgery,* Vol. 20, No. 7, pp. 949–952, ISSN 0960-8923.

[81] Silver, HJ., Torquati, A., Jensen, GL., Richards, WO. (2006). Weight, dietary and physical exercises behaviors two years after gastric bypass. *Obesity Surgery,* Vol. 16, pp. 859-864, ISSN 0960-8923.

[82] Taheri, E., Saedisomeolia, A., Djalali, M., Qorbani, M., Madani Civi, M. (2012). The relationship between serum 25-hydroxy vitamin D concentration and obesity in type 2 diabetic patients and healthy subjects. *Journal of Diabetes and Metabolic Disorders,* Vol. 11, No. 1, pp. 16, ISSN 2251-6581.

[83] Toh, SY., Zarshenas, N., Jorgensen, J. (2009). Prevalence of nutrient deficiencies in bariatric patients. *Nutrition,* Vol. 25, No. 11-12, pp. 1150-1156, ISSN 0899-9007.

[84] Trabulsi, J., Schoeller, DA. (2001). Evaluation of dietary assessment instruments against doubly labeled water, a biomarker of habitual energy intake. *American Journal of Physiology: Endocrinology and Metabolism,* Vol. 281, No. 5, pp. E891-E899, ISSN 0193-1849.

[85] Togo, P., Osler, M., Sørensen, TI., Heitmann, BL. (2001). Food intake patterns and body mass index in observational studies. *International Journal of Obesity and Related Metabolic Disorders,* Vol. 25, No. 12, pp. 1741-1751, ISSN 0307-0565.

Chapter 3

Complications of Bariatric Surgery

Young Kim and Peter F. Crookes

Additional information is available at the end of the chapter

http://dx.doi.org/10.5772/58920

1. Introduction

The widespread adoption of bariatric surgery as a major therapeutic option for patients with severe obesity, especially when associated with serious metabolic comorbidities, is a relatively recent phenomenon and has inevitably resulted in large numbers of patients who may present to physicians who have not had specific training in this field of medicine. Bariatric surgery has also become one of the targets of the medical tourist industry, where patients can choose to go abroad to get surgery which may cost only a fraction of what it would cost in the USA. In the event of a problem occurring after the patients return home, they will most likely present to an adjacent Emergency Room, often with little knowledge or documentation of what they had and why. The purpose of this chapter is to highlight the major things that can go wrong after bariatric surgery. The term *complications* is generally restricted to situations where surgery has caused an identifiable disease process, for example abdominal sepsis, bowel obstruction, or hemorrhage or malnutrition. In addition there are other adverse effects of surgery which are not true complications but which nevertheless result in a dissatisfied patient, for example, weight regain after initial success, the presence of large floppy folds of skin, or persistent GI symptoms of nausea and vomiting. Although major complications after contemporary surgery are relatively rare, they do consume a great deal of healthcare resources to investigate and treat. They not only cause symptoms and anxiety for the patient and family, but also may be a major source of stress for the bariatric team especially if hostility in the doctor-patient relationship leads to a lawsuit. It is therefore especially important that all physicians are familiar with the major forms of bariatric surgery and the spectrum of complications to which the surgery may give rise.

Early recognition of complications and prompt treatment or referral to a specialist center is the most important way to minimize their ill effects. This chapter will focus on the definition, recognition and range of treatment options for the major complications of the principal bariatric procedures in contemporary practice, based on our own experience in a tertiary

INTECH
open science | open minds

© 2014 The Author(s). Licensee InTech. This chapter is distributed under the terms of the Creative Commons Attribution License (http://creativecommons.org/licenses/by/3.0), which permits unrestricted use, distribution, and reproduction in any medium, provided the original work is properly cited.

referral center as well as major reports in the recent literature. The details of individual operations are covered in other chapters in this book and will not be recapitulated here.

The simplest way to classify complications is to stratify them according to the time since surgery, generally into three major time periods

- Perioperative (the first month)
- Intermediate (the first 12 months)
- Late (one or more years after the surgery)

Although there is some overlap, the spectrum of complications in each time period is sufficiently distinct to consider them separately. Perioperative complications are always managed primarily by the surgeon but later events may be managed by the primary care physician or other specialists.

2. Perioperative complications

Responsibility for recognition of perioperative complications always rests with the operating surgeon. There is evidence to suggest that complications are more frequent after open bariatric surgery than laparoscopic procedures, but some of these differences are undoubtedly related to the fact that until recently, open procedures were used for the most high risk patients who were felt unsuitable for laparoscopy [1].

Perioperative complications can be classified simply into Cardiorespiratory problems which include myocardial infarction (MI), pulmonary embolism (PE) and/or Deep Venous Thrombosis (DVT), Surgical problems (leak or stenosis of the anastomosis, bleeding, and incisional problems) and issues related to the underlying comorbidities, such as the management of CPAP machines or diabetic, transplant or antipsychotic medications.

2.1. The moribund patient

The most alarming situation confronting the surgeon in the early postoperative phase is the patient who deteriorates within a very short time, usually with tachycardia and hypotension and hypoxia, prompting the need for intubation and administration of pressors. Although rare, it is important to reach a diagnosis quickly or the patient will rapidly go into an irreversible decline. Most such cases are accounted for by a quartet of conditions – pulmonary embolism, myocardial infarction, bleeding and sepsis (usually from a leak) – which must be immediately considered before thinking of more esoteric conditions. When this state occurs years after surgery, it is generally thought to be due to sepsis, but micronutrient deficiencies, particularly of Thiamine (Vitamin B1) have occasionally been incriminated in the pathogenesis of this critical state. This is discussed in the section of late complications.

2.2. Cardiorespiratory complications

All of these typically present with chest pain or discomfort, shortage of breath, anxiety and tachycardia. Perioperative *myocardial infarction* is high on the list in a patient with a known history of coronary artery disease especially if it has required stenting or coronary artery bypass grafting in the past [2]. Typically such a patient is on antiplatelet medication such as aspirin and clopidrogel (Plavix) which has been discontinued a week before surgery and not restarted because of the risk of creating bleeding. A patient with chest pain after surgery should have immediate 12-lead EKG and measurement of troponin levels. Elevated troponin levels or the presence of ST elevation should prompt immediate cardiology consultation as early clot dissolution or re-stenting can limit the myocardial damage. Surgeons are naturally worried about resumption of antiplatelet agents soon after surgery, but a reasonable compromise for patients who have stopped antiplatelet therapy is to resume aspirin in the recovery ward, usually by suppository, and restart other agents such as Clopidrogel a week later when the risk of bleeding should have receded.

2.2.1. Venous thromboembolism (VTE)

Many factors commonly found in the bariatric population predispose to VTE, including the mechanical effects of superobesity, prior VTE history, obesity hypoventilation syndrome, use of hormonal therapy, immobility and venous stasis disease. Most surgeons advocate both mechanical and chemical modes of prophylaxis in the perioperative period, and many also recommend continuation of heparin therapy for several weeks after discharge [3].

Pulmonary embolism (PE) is very rare after laparoscopic bariatric surgery, but is a significant risk in patients undergoing open surgery or who have surgery for complications especially in the context of a prolonged hospital stay. The overall incidence has been estimated at 0.9% but fatalities are estimated at 0.03% [4, 5].

Patients with a past history of Venous Thromboembolism are at greatest risk, especially if anticoagulation was stopped in preparation for the surgery. The key features are hypoxia and hypotension and tachypnea, and the patients are often anxious, sometimes causing the symptoms to be dismissed as "hyperventilation syndrome." The patient may be cyanosed with cool sweating extremities. An EKG and chest x ray will be done immediately, chiefly to exclude other serious pathology such as MI or tension pneumothorax. Massive pulmonary embolism may be so rapidly fatal that no confirmation of diagnosis is possible, and the majority of deaths that occur in contemporary practice from pulmonary embolism happen within an hour of the onset of the symptoms.

A patient with these features suspected of pulmonary embolism needs a rapid diagnosis. To begin anticoagulation or more invasive treatment such as fibrinolytic therapy shortly after major surgery requires more than strong clinical suspicion. A bedside echocardiogram may show right ventricular dilation, and commonly a chest CT angiogram will show significant filling defects. CT scanning is immediately available in most facilities and gives information about massive embolism comparable to pulmonary angiography. CT confirmation is sufficient to justify invasive therapy such as anticoagulation or thrombolysis. There is no time to wait for biomarkers such as BNP and D-Dimer or the results of a nuclear medicine (V/Q) scan. The therapeutic options depend on the severity of the situation and include anticoagulation, fibrinolytic agents, catheter directed thrombolysis and pulmonary embolectomy. Insertion of a caval filter pending the introduction of anticoagulation is often recommended in patients with new-onset deep venous thrombosis. However, prophylactic insertion of caval filters in patients with significant risk factors is more controversial and is generally not recommended [6].

Deep venous thrombosis may occur in up to 1.3% of patients after open or laparoscopic bariatric surgery. Despite the enhanced mobility after laparoscopic surgery, the incidence of DVT may not be reduced as much as expected because the benefit of early motility may be offset by the tendency of pneumoperitoneum to promote DVT. All major bariatric surgeons are agreed that a combination of mechanical (sequential calf compression devices or anti-embolism compressive stockings) and chemical (either unfractionated or low-molecular-weight heparin) should be employed prophylactically. Some surgeons advocate continuation of heparin after discharge for up to 30 days [7]. Detection on purely clinical grounds is often difficult because of the physical dimensions of the patient's legs, but asymmetrical edema or leg pain should encourage the surgeon to search for DVT, usually by duplex scanning.

2.3. Bleeding

Postoperative bleeding rarely presents with such a catastrophic deterioration, but is associated with tachycardia, oliguria and falling hemoglobin (Hb) level. Obvious risk factors include the need for preoperative anticoagulation, or surgery rendered difficult by adhesions or limited visibility [8].

In a patient who is hemodynamically stable there is time for confirmatory checks to ensure a downward trend in Hb, because sometimes a patient with tachycardia or hypotension for other reasons will be administered large volumes of IV fluid causing the Hb to drop transiently by hemodilution. Postoperative bleeding may occur into the peritoneal cavity or into the GI tract [9-11].

In the former, the only evidence of bleeding is indirect, and is inferred when the patient shows general signs of hemorrhage including tachycardia, oliguria, hypotension and falling Hb levels. If the recent surgery was known to be difficult the source may be easy to suspect: typical sites are the dissection round the cardia, the omentum, or inadvertent injury to the liver or spleen. Unless the patient is becoming hemodynamically unstable, most surgeons would recommend transfusion of up to two units of packed red cells, since most of these bleeding sites are self limiting. A patient who continues to bleed as evidenced by persistent tachycardia and failure of the Hb to come up and stay up appropriately after transfusion is most safely managed by return to the operating room. Repeat laparoscopy generally shows a substantial amount of clot in the peritoneal cavity, but in the majority of cases the bleeding has stopped.

GI Bleeding is associated with the general signs of hemorrhage but there is also vomiting of blood or passage of blood per rectum. The source of GI bleeding is almost always from the staple or suture lines. Other sources of GI bleeding seen in non-bariatric practice such as

http://dx.doi.org/10.5772/58920

esophageal varices or peptic ulceration are largely irrelevant to the bariatric surgery patient. The three potential sources are from the Gastrojejunal (GJ) anastomosis, from the Jejuno-jejunostomy (JJ), or from the long staple line in the bypassed stomach (Figure 1). GI bleeding is more serious than intraperitoneal bleeding because the low pH of the stomach inhibits the coagulation process and the bleed is less likely to be self limiting. Therefore, a hemodynamically unstable patient with a GI bleed should be rapidly resuscitated and returned to the operating room immediately. It is important to have an experienced upper GI endoscopist available. If, on putting in the laparoscope, the remnant stomach is seen to be very distended, the source is likely in the suture line of the bypassed stomach. The stomach should be opened and the clot evacuated. A continuous running suture to under-run the staple line is all that is required to stop the hemorrhage and it is not necessary to open the staple line itself.

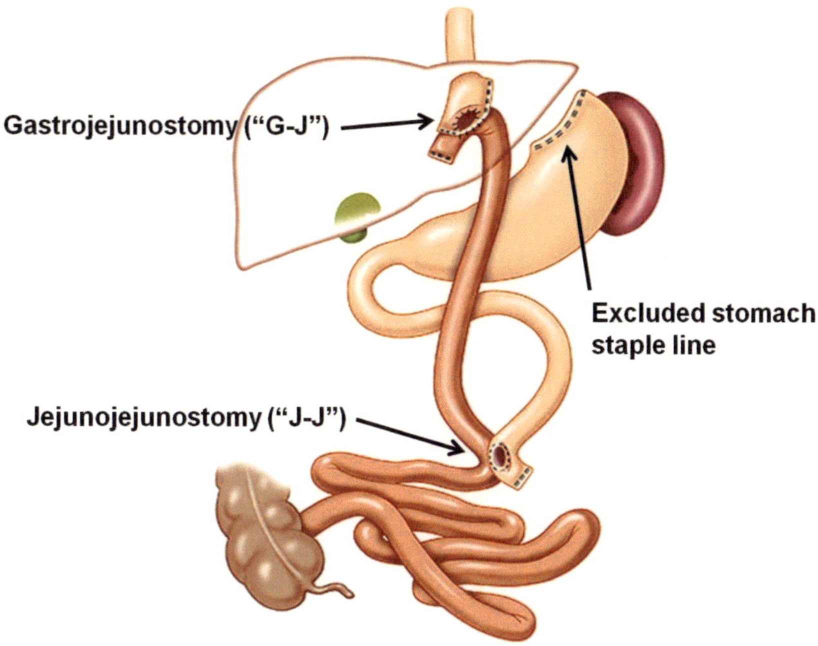

Figure 1. Diagram illustrating the potential sites of GI bleeding after gastric bypass.

Bleeding from the GJ or JJ anastomosis is more problematic and may require intraoperative upper GI endoscopy to identify the site. The bariatric surgeon who is also a skilled endoscopist has the advantage of knowing the anatomy of the reconstruction, but in typical practice, a gastroenterologist or other GI surgical colleague will be helpful during return to the operating room. Extreme gentleness of manipulation and limitation of air insufflation is essential. If the operating surgeon sees that the remnant stomach is not distended, the Roux limb should be clamped with long grasping forceps while the endoscopist inspects the gastric pouch and GJ anastomosis. This limits the diffuse dilation of the entire GI tract by the endoscopist. If bleeding is identified, it may be clipped if it is from a single site and accessible to the endoscopist, or the surgeon can reinforce it with a full thickness layer of running monofilament absorbable suture. If there is no blood in the gastric pouch and the anastomosis is not bleeding, the bowel should be clamped just distal to the JJ anastomosis and the scope advanced distally. Bleeding of sufficient magnitude to justify return to the OR often causes large amounts of clot into the jejunum which can then become obstructed [12].

In this case, the surgeon can make a small enterotomy and evacuate the clot because manipulating the anastomosis in this situation may cause the whole reconstruction to fall apart. If there are no big clots visible, the operating surgeon can assist the passage of the scope by pushing the jejunum up over the scope rather like putting the foot into a long sock. In this way the JJ anastomosis may be reached with a conventional endoscope.

In addition to physical control of bleeding, either endoscopically or surgically, an intravenous infusion of pantoprazole (4-8mg /hour) is recommended to produce sustained reduction of gastric acidity and facilitate the clotting process within the upper GI tract.

2.4. Leakage and sepsis

This is the commonest and most feared early complication, and the one most directly related to surgical technique. Leakage can occur from any suture or staple line after gastric bypass or sleeve gastrectomy or even from unrecognized perforation at the time of adjustable band insertion. In practice the two most common sites to leak are the staple line after sleeve gastrectomy (where the incidence is 1-3%) and the GJ anastomosis after gastric bypass where the incidence is in the 1% range. In revisional bariatric surgery, the risks are much higher and the incidence may be ten times higher than in first time cases.

There are two major forms of presentation: early and delayed. Very early leaks (while the patient is still in hospital) present with severe abdominal pain and signs of peritonitis because there has been no time for localization. They are generally anxious or agitated. Early leaks are presumed to be due to a technical problem in anastomotic construction such as misfiring of a stapler or inadequate suture technique. In contrast, leaks presenting in the second week, after the patient has left hospital and is taking a liquid diet, present more like intra-abdominal abscess with fever and often shoulder tip pain. These later leaks may be due to ischemia of the suture line. The development of the perforation is sufficiently gradual for some localization by omentum and adjacent structures to have occurred.

Sometimes the symptoms of chest and shoulder discomfort and shortage of breath predominate, leading to a workup to rule out pulmonary embolism. The surgeon should be aware that statistically such a patient is much more likely to have a leak than a PE and should be investigated accordingly. We often quote an old aphorism which states *"the lung is the mirror of the abdomen"* meaning that pulmonary symptoms are merely reflecting some pathologic process in the upper abdomen. There is a strong temptation for the surgeon to be in denial when faced with a patient with pain and tachycardia after surgery. Psychologically it easier to attribute the clinical picture to some less critical factor such as bowel distention, pneumonia, or narcotic dependency, but the surgeon should make strenuous efforts to detect a leak before considering these other putative causes.

http://dx.doi.org/10.5772/58920

Large leaks may be detected by a contrast swallow but the sensitivity is low and the study may not be available out of hours. It is easier to obtain an abdominal CT scan with oral and IV contrast, which will most likely show signs of bubbles of free air and extravasated contrast (Figure 2).

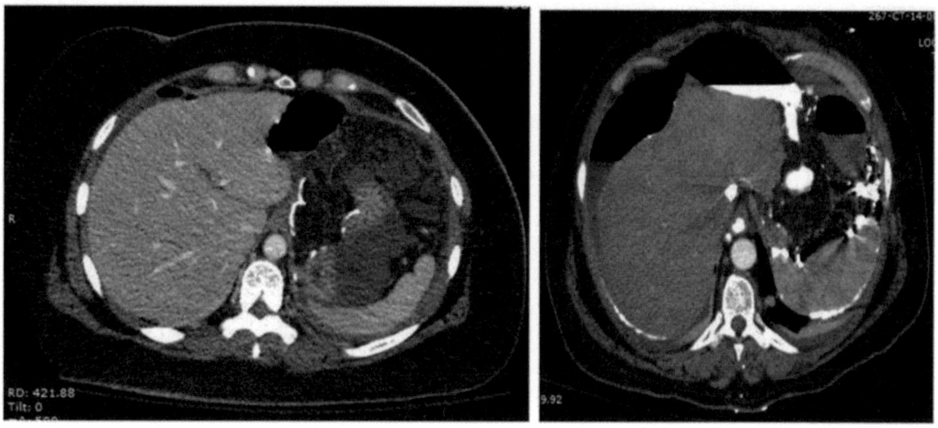

Figure 2. (a) CT Scan showing early leakage after gastric bypass. Note the small pocket of air and the small amount of fluid over the liver, (b) A more extreme example with a greater degree of free air and fluid after a gastric bypass revision. Note that the patient has residual barium many years after a prior leakage after a laparoscopic adjustable gastric band

Not every leak requires an automatic return to the operating room [13]. The range of therapeutic options for leaks includes simple drainage under CT guidance, stenting, clipping or return to the OR for resuture or revision of the anastomosis, and placement of accurate drains. It may be very difficult to identify the precise site of the leak at surgery because of the surrounding tissue distortion and adhesions. When the leak is located, resuture alone is rarely successful. Placement of accurate drainage is helpful, because if subsequently it is possible to seal the leak endoscopically by clipping or deployment of a stent, there will not be a contained pocket of contaminated contents. One promising approach is actually to insert a drain into the leak endoscopically and provide internal drainage. Typically a biliary stent is employed for this purpose. As the leak heals and the extraluminal cavity shrinks, the stent gets pushed more and more into the lumen.

Leaks from sleeve gastrectomy, regardless of whether or not it was combined with a duodenal switch, are harder to manage. Their characteristics are becoming well recognized as sleeve gastrectomy increases in popularity almost exponentially. These leaks almost always occur at the most proximal portion of the staple line. This is partly because it is a watershed area with relatively poor blood supply, and also because there is frequently a relative obstruction in the mid body portion of the stomach as the narrow gastric sleeve traverses the incisura angularis. High pressure in the proximal portion of the gastric body promotes leakage of the staple line and retards healing because the leak offers the path of least resistance for ingested liquids. Gastric juice and bile as well as swallowed saliva are present, thus patients leaking from SG tend to be sicker than patients leaking from gastric bypass. The same principles of treatment are necessary, but in addition the surgeon must ensure that there is no distal resistance in the narrow stomach. Insertion of a stent may straighten out this tight angulation, and it may in fact be the way in which stents promote healing, since they do not produce a water tight seal. When conservative treatments fail, operative approaches include either transecting the stomach above the leak, which usually entails an esophago-jejunostomy, or bringing up a Roux limb to cover the leak as described by Baltasar et al [14].

In large series reported from specialist centers, leaks after laparoscopic gastric bypass have an incidence of 1% or less, and after sleeve gastrectomy the reported risks are in the range of 1-3%. It is likely that in routine clinical practice these rates are higher than what is reported because of publication bias, since units with higher complication rates are less likely to publish the results.

In future, advances in endoscopic technology may permit better endoscopic clipping and suturing, but these methods at present are rarely successful, mostly because the underlying conditions-tissue ischemia and high intraluminal pressure – have not been dealt with.

2.4.1. Newer operations

Gastric plication has gained some popularity in a few centers because it is potentially reversible and avoids the need for actual resection. Patients presenting with problems after these kinds of procedures are usually well informed and it is generally easy to find literature reports to elucidate confusing clinical pictures [15-17].

2.5. Wound complications

Wound problems after laparoscopic surgery are very rare, unless a circular stapler was used to create the GJ anastomosis, in which case it is difficult to protect the wound edge from the contaminated stapler as it is extracted from the body. After open surgery, in contrast, wound infections are quite common, because the great depth of subcutaneous fat permits the exudation of serum or blood which leads to infection when the surgical wound is categorized as contaminated. Quite often it only appears after the patient is discharged and it is important to be vigilant in the early postoperative course for signs of wound infection, which include erythema, induration, "peau d'orange" changes in the skin, and actual fluctuation. Although wound infection is traditionally treated by simple incision and drainage, and subsequently by frequent packing or continuous low pressure suction, it is a very long drawn out process that may require weeks or months to heal by secondary intention and increases the chance of subsequent incisional herniation.

2.6. Other rare complications

2.6.1. Mesenteric venous thrombosis

This serious complication has been described after both gastric bypass and sleeve gastrectomy, and it presents with non-specific findings of abdominal pain, nausea, vomiting and low grade fever and are initially suspected to have a leak. The finding of thrombosis of the mesenteric and portal veins is readily apparent on CT scanning. Milder cases respond to systemic anticoagulation, but some require intraportal administration of thrombolytics, and occasionally bowel resection or splenectomy is required. It is thought to represent a manifestation of the hypercoagulable state, and a significant percentage have a history of venous thromboembolism in the past or current oral contraceptive use [18].

2.6.2. Rhabdomyolysis

One rare but immediately recognizable early complication is rhabdomyolysis of the gluteal muscles, which presents with severe pain in the buttocks or legs. It appears to be the result of pressure necrosis of the muscles, initially by unrelieved pressure on the operating table, and amplified by edema and swelling within the gluteal muscle compartment [19]. If unrecognized, extensive skin necrosis overlying the gluteal muscles may develop (Figure 3).

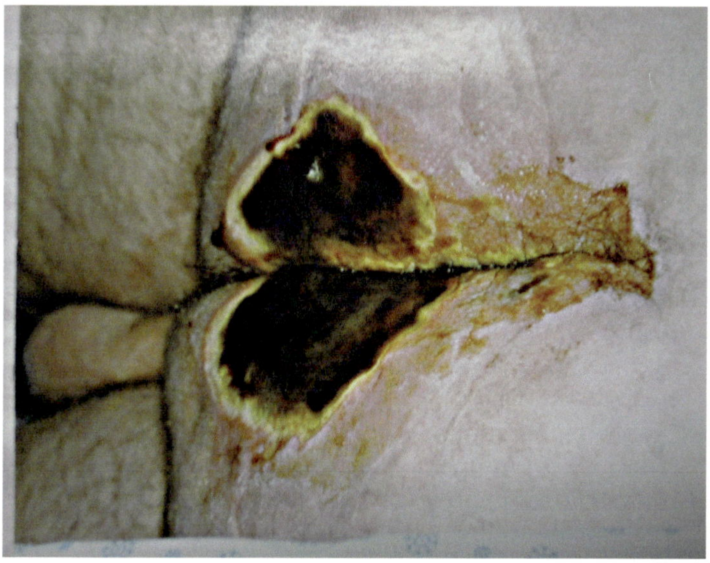

Figure 3. Extensive skin necrosis of the buttocks as a consequence of gluteal muscle rhabdomyolysis

It is most often noted in superobese males with diabetes and central obesity who have a prolonged operative procedure. The swollen muscle can compress the sciatic nerve or its roots and can release myoglobin and cause renal failure. The diagnosis is clinched by very elevated creatine kinase (CK) levels. After uncomplicated surgery, CK levels may be up to 1200 units/l in the first 48 hours, but rhabdomyolysis causes values of 30, 000 units/l or even more. It is important not to dismiss the symptoms as due to "arthritis" or its cutaneous manifestation as a decubitus ulcer, because immediate decompression may limit the loss of muscle and the extent of nerve injury. Since it was first described, widespread attention to careful padding on the operating table and limiting the duration of surgery in high risk patients have helped prevent the condition.

2.6.3. Nerve injuries

In a similar way, compression of peripheral nerves such as the ulnar or common peroneal nerve may occur because of positioning on the operating table during a lengthy operation. Traction injury to the brachial plexus may occur if the angle of the outstretched arms on the operating table is greater than 90°. When the table is put into reverse Trendelenburg position, the body tends to slide down the table and increase this angle, leading to a traction injury causing dysesthesia and motor weakness in the arms and hands. When a patient reports such findings after surgery, it is important to document the time of onset and to obtain neurological consultation, because persistence of the symptoms may prompt the patient to file a lawsuit, especially if there was a perception that the complaint was not taken seriously [20-22].

3. Intermediate term complications: the first year

After recovery from surgery, the initial rapid rate of weight loss (often 0.5kg per day at first) levels off so that the body weight has reached a plateau by the end of the first year. Several issues may arise during this time, some of them surgical problems and others related to comorbidities of difficulties in adjusting to the new state of the GI tract.

3.1. Small Bowel Obstruction

Small bowel obstruction can follow any abdominal operation. In practice, it is extremely rare after a purely gastric operation such as SG or LAGB. The potential causes are more numerous after operations involving intestinal rearrangement. In the first few weeks, trapping of a loop of bowel may occur in a laparoscopic port site, or an umbilical or incisional hernia that was not repaired at the time of the bypass. This is why it is recommended not to dissect omentum out of abdominal wall hernias at the time of bariatric surgery unless the hernia is to be formally repaired as part of the case. *Internal hernias* may occur in three situations after bypass (Figure 4). The commonest is underneath the free edge of the mesentery of the biliopancreatic limb. There is a free cut edge of mesentery in the Roux limb in addition, but herniation under this limb is rare if it is antecolic. If it is retrocolic, the opening in the transverse mesocolon or the space between the mesentery and the mesocolon (Petersen's space) are also potential sites for herniation. Most surgeons close these defects at the time of surgery but as weight is lost and the mesentery becomes thinner, it is possible for the defect to open months or years later. They are commoner after laparoscopic gastric bypass than in open operations, presumably because there are fewer adhesions after laparoscopic surgery [23].

The investigation of choice is the CT scan, because it will make the diagnosis, identify any abdominal wall defects trapping the bowel, and has the highest specificity and sensitivity for detecting an internal hernia, the so-called "mesenteric swirl" sign [24].

It is often possible to correct these situations laparoscopically because the adhesions are much less numerous that after open surgery. In addition to hernia as a cause of small bowel obstruction, adhesions especially to the J-J anastomosis may cause mechanical obstruction.

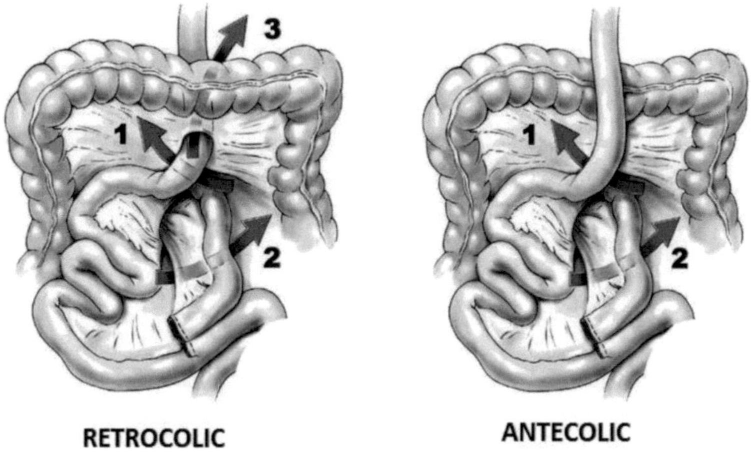

In the retrocolic approach, a loop of bowel can get trapped between the Roux limb mesentery and the transverse mesocolon (1, sometimes called Peterson's space), in the opening of the transverse mesocolon (2) or in the mesenteric opening of the biliopancreatic limb (3). In the more common antecolic approach, there is no opening in the transverse mesocolon and hernia behind the Roux limb is less common.

Figure 4. Three potential sites for internal herniation after Roux Y gastric bypass.

A unique form of small bowel obstruction may affect patients with the DS, when the biliopancreatic limb becomes obstructed (Figure 5). This presents with very severe central abdominal pain though normal bowel movements may be preserved: it may progress rapidly to intestinal ischemia and gangrene if not decompressed because it is a closed-loop obstruction. Since it is not accessible to nasogastric suction or endoscopic decompression, it requires urgent surgery. Consequently a patient presenting with severe abdominal pain after DS should have an immediate CT scan of the abdomen to check for dilated loops of the biliopancreatic limb.

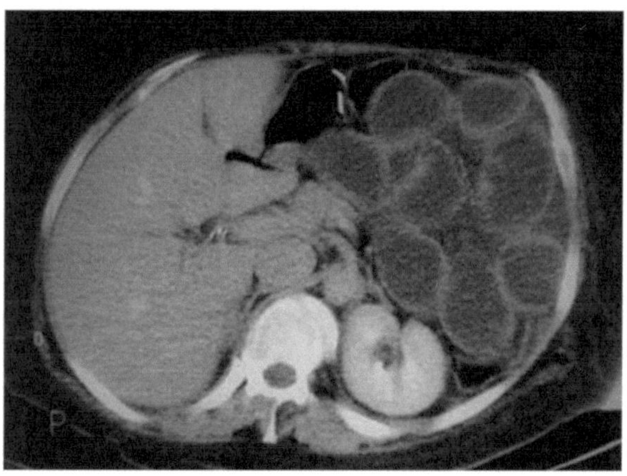

Figure 5. CT scan showing obstruction to the biliopancreatic limb after duodenal switch. Note the dilated non-opacified loops of bowel in the left upper quadrant.

3.1.1. GI dysfunction

3.1.1.1. Stricture and ulcer

The narrow gastric pouch after GBP or SG is very restrictive at the beginning, and patients can usually tolerate only clear liquids in small quantities at first. Patients are usually given written instructions to guide the gradual increase in the quantity and range of foods they can tolerate. Patients who do not receive or who do not understand such instruction have a high incidence of vomiting postoperatively. Many patients will experience a few episodes of vomiting if they relax the vigilance with which they increase their dietary intake, and some vomiting is probably inevitable as they learn how to cope with a sensation of fullness, which is a novel experience for most bariatric patients. However, in well instructed and supported patients, it should be rare. Rather than berate the patient for failure of compliance, or attribute vomiting to persistence of a psychological compulsion to eat large quantities quickly, the physician should consider organic causes, namely a stricture [25].

Some degree of stricturing of the GJ anastomosis is common, and usually resolves with time (less than 3 months) and can be managed by going back to softer or liquid foods. A more severe stricture may be due to an ulcer at the anastomosis, and the physician should inquire about consumption of NSAID or large pills, or resumption of smoking. Endoscopy typically reveals an ulcer with visible suture material or staples (Figure 6). A fibrous stricture may develop later Such strictures generally respond to one or two dilations (Figure 7). Patients are often put on proton pump inhibitors (PPI) empirically to help reduce recurrence.

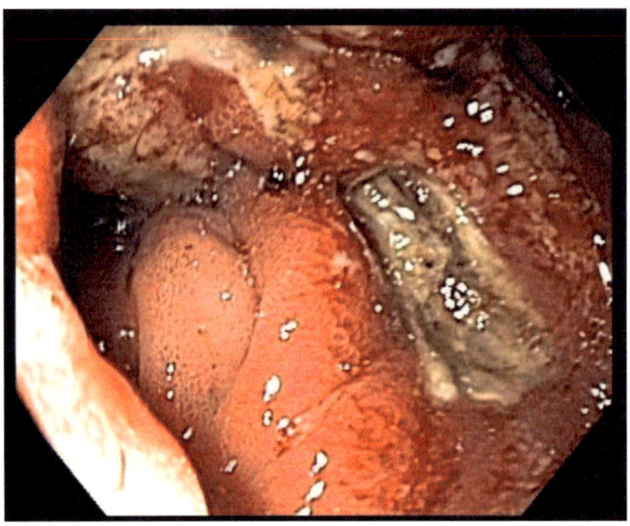

Figure 6. Ulcer at the G-J anastomosis visible on endoscopy

Severe or refractory strictures usually are caused by ulcers which do not heal, and are more frequent in smokers. Other contributing factors are consumption of over the counter medica-

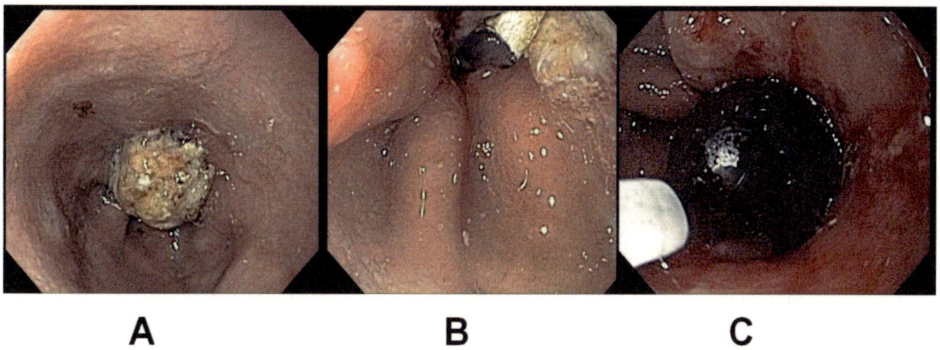

Figure 7. Stricture at the G-J anastomosis (a) obscured by food particles, (b) after removal of food material and (c) during dilation

tions for headaches or other painful conditions. This persistent ulceration may also have an ischemic component, in which case it appears to respond well to reoperation when the gastric pouch is shortened and the weight loss permits the Roux limb to be easily brought up to the stomach without tension.

3.1.1.2. Gastroesophageal reflux disease (GERD)

In general, patients with pre-existing GERD experience a profound improvement in reflux symptoms after GBP. This is largely because only a tiny fraction of the acid secreting mucosa has any access to the esophagus. Persistence or recurrence of reflux symptoms suggests that the pouch is too large, or that a hiatal hernia was undetected or uncorrected. If reflux symptoms occur for the first time after an interval of months or years postoperatively, it suggests the presence of a gastro-gastric fistula (see below).

The situation is quite different after operations such as the Sleeve Gastrectomy and duodenal switch. In both operations there is a notable incidence of persistent or new-onset GERD [26, 27]. It may be caused by overzealous resection of the proximal fundus including the gastric sling fibers, thus weakening the lower esophageal sphincter. Failure to identify and repair a hiatal hernia has also been incriminated. Finally, the configuration of the sleeve tends to produce a sharp angle at the incisura angularis which acts as a relative obstruction, thus promoting reflux. GERD after DS or SG is problematic because sometimes PPI medications are of limited efficacy or limited by side effects such as diarrhea. The most efficacious way of controlling this is to convert the situation to a Roux Y gastric bypass by transecting the stomach high up, leaving a pouch the size of a typical GBP. This effectively abolishes GERD and disconnects the esophagus from all but the smallest quantities of acid.

3.1.1.3. Constipation and diarrhea

Operations confined to the stomach, namely SG and LAGB, rarely affect bowel function. Gastric bypass typically causes constipation, which can be managed by regular stool softeners and over the counter remedies. Severe constipation is common in patients who take continuous narcotic pain medications, but otherwise it may be a manifestation of Small Bowel Bacterial Overgrowth (SIBO). This is diagnosed by a breath test in response to ingested glucose and often responds to a course of Rifaximin, a non-absorbable antibiotic. Diarrhea after gastric bypass is rare and the stool should be checked for *Clostridium Difficile* before resorting to symptomatic treatment. Most such cases are managed by dietary adjustments such as avoidance of lactose containing products. Anecdotal evidence supports the use of probiotics in this situation. Intractable diarrhea is a terribly crippling social problem and patients will usually be referred to a gastroenterologist. In a person with no prior history of diarrhea and no evidence of infective colitis, the cause is rarely clear, and has been attributed to such entities as vagal nerve damage or bacterial overgrowth. Colonoscopy is useful to look for other forms of colitis, and long term somatostatin analogues may be helpful. We have had several patients with refractory and crippling diarrhea in which the only measure that proved of value was reversal of the gastric bypass.

The bowel habit after DS and other malabsorptive operations is typically characterized by 2-3 soft and malodorous stools daily, depending on the intake of fat or refined carbohydrates. More than this suggests either lack of dietary compliance, or bacterial overgrowth, or both. When these symptoms occur in an otherwise asymptomatic patient, we have found empirically that low-dose Metronidazole (250mg bid) produces significantly improvement. The physician should be alert to the possibility that it may be a manifestation of serious malnutrition, as discussed below.

3.1.1.4. Hyperinsulinemic hypoglycemia

Hypoglycemia associated with excessive insulin secretion, has been reported after GBP, and has been attributed to nesidiobastosis [28, 29], possibly mediated by the effect of GLP-1 on the pancreas.

It presents with episodes of altered mental status associated with profound hypoglycemia, and seems to occur in those who were non-diabetic at the time of surgery. T here is recent evidence that the phenomenon is much more prevalent than suggested by the literature, consisting as it does of small case series. A recent presentation to the American Diabetic Association described prospective continuous blood sugar monitoring after both GBP and DS and found hypoglycemic episodes, most of them asymptomatic, averaging 42 minutes per day after GBP and 85 minutes per day after DS, whereas none of the controls experienced hypoglycemia.

Any patient reporting symptoms suggestive of episodic hypoglycemia should be provided with a home glucose monitor and instructed in it use over a period of several days, to document if hypoglycemia is actually occurring. This simple step often eliminates it as a diagnosis. Typically, fasting blood glucose is normal, but drops occur after food. It thus resembles an extreme form of reactive hypoglycemia. The workup for hypoglycemia is complex, and since the episodes can cause serious mental status changes, they may have very serious consequences, for example if the patient is driving a vehicle or operating machinery. Hence prompt referral to an endocrinologist is recommended. Dietary adjustment to increase protein and reduce carbohydrate consumption may help, as may administration of diazoxide or even streptozotocin.

Some of these patients have been found to respond to distal pancreatectomy, but we have had several patients who were much improved by the much simpler technique of shortening of the Roux limb by anastomosing it to the biliopancreatic limb more proximally.

3.2. Surgical complications specific to individual bariatric operations

3.2.1. Laparoscopic adjustable gastric banding – slippage and erosion

The band in this procedure typically sits immediately below the gastroesophageal junction. It can gradually slip downwards and allow a large portion of fundus or the body of the stomach to prolapse through it, which can result in compartmentalization of the stomach with outlet obstruction [30]. Such patients have severe vomiting, dysphagia and gastroesophageal reflux. This is a serious situation where there is a risk of gastric necrosis or perforation. The band is immediately deflated in the emergency room and the patient should be taken to the operating room without delay. Most surgeons would simply remove the band and allow the stomach to recover. In delayed cases there may be necrosis of a large portion of the stomach, in which case it is safest to excise the ischemic portion, insert a feeding tube in the distal remnant stomach, and a drainage tube the remaining viable fundus and then do a planned reconstruction a few months later when the patient is in stable condition and there are no nutritional or infective problems. The reconstructive options are to do a simple gastro-gastrostomy or to convert to a Roux-Y gastric bypass.

Band erosion typically presents more slowly. Here the band erodes gradually into the lumen of the stomach. This presents with loss of any sense of restriction, weight gain, and tracking of infection from the stomach presenting as infection of the site of the subcutaneous port [31]. It is readily diagnosed on endoscopy, when the stained plastic of the band will be readily seen near the cardia. It is less common in recent years with the adoption of the *pars flaccida* technique rather than the perigastric technique. Bands which are almost completely eroded into the stomach may be removed endoscopically by cutting the band, pulling it into the lumen of the stomach, transecting the tubing, and withdrawing it through the mouth. This avoids the need to dissect the dense adhesions and scar that have sealed off the band from the peritoneal cavity [32].

3.2.2. Malabsorptive operations (Biliopancreatic Diversion and Duodenal Switch)

The principal surgical complications especially found after malabsorptive operations include

1. Biliopancreatic limb obstruction, discussed above
2. Protein-energy and other forms of malnutrition, discussed in the following section.
3. Severe and refractory gastroesophageal reflux. This has emerged as a leading cause of morbidity after any kind of sleeve gastrectomy, whether as a stand-alone operation or as part of a duodenal switch.

4. Long term complications

4.1. Malnutrition

Various forms of nutritional deficiency can develop after bariatric surgery, and the operations which produce the greatest weight loss tend to produce more nutritional problems. Modern bariatric operations are much safer in this regard than the original Jejunoileal bypass operations, but the risk remains. Deficiencies are least prominent after LAGB and SG, and greatest after BPD and DS [33, 34]. Long term follow up with regular monitoring of weight and nutritional status are designed to identify potential problems which can be addressed before a serious clinical problem develops.

Laboratory assessment of nutritional status has become more standardized in recent years and guidelines from numerous professional societies have been published. Most programs agree on the need for annual monitoring of nutritional parameters, ideally through the operating surgeon's office or the patient's primary care doctor. These annual visits include documentation of the patient's intake of food, vitamins and nutritional supplements, and measurement of a range of laboratory values as indicated in the table. Those who are lost to follow-up or whose psychosocial equilibrium is disrupted are at greater risk of nutritional deficiency. The first step in caring for any patient who presents for follow up to a different physician, or after a long interval of neglect, is to review the nature of the procedure, make a careful assessment of the current eating practices, usually with the help of a dietitian, and obtain the above laboratory values. Physicians should recognize that malnourished patients are often reluctant to seek help because of fear of weight regain, and often only come to attention when some other medical crisis occurs. It is therefore important to detect when a nutritional deficiency is something that requires surgical revision of the procedure and when it is simply a matter of education and compliance in taking additional supplements [35].

Protein Energy malnutrition is a consequence of either inadequate intake or inadequate absorption. Poor intake is usually associated with restrictive operations which cause anorexia, physical restriction of oral intake, or both. A history of extremely limited intake, frequent dysphagia and regurgitation of food particles or saliva, is common. Patients will frequently describe "bringing up foam" because the esophagus fills with saliva which then is displaced proximally when food or liquid is ingested. Maladaptive eating patterns may involve so-called "slider" foods such as ice cream and soups, often high in calories and fat but low in protein, or may be described as bizarre or crazy, as in the obsession for crushed ice.

In contrast, patients with malabsorption may appear to eat well but will often report diarrhea or steatorrhea. In both cases, there may be generalized weakness and fatiguability, and edema, which in severe cases is not limited to the ankles and feet but may be obvious even in the back and chest wall. Serum albumin is often very low, less than 3.0 g/l and in severest cases less than 2.0 g/l. These extreme cases are more frequently observed after malabsorptive operations but can occur after any bariatric operation.

Intensive dietary supervision and monitoring by the dietitian, and careful follow up to assess the effect of these interventions are essential. If the underlying reason can be corrected,

http://dx.doi.org/10.5772/58920

restoration is frequently achieved. Such factors as lack of awareness, divorce, unemployment, financial crisis, psychiatric illness, or development of other addictions may all contribute. A dietitian, psychologist, social worker, psychiatrist and counselor may all be necessary to help get the patient back on track. Sometimes the nutritional problems persist despite removal of any barriers to compliance. In this situation, consideration must be given to some kind of revision or even reversal of the procedure.

4.2. Revision of bariatric procedures for malnutrition

In this section, we distinguish the need for revision to correct malnutrition from some other clinical situations in which revision may be important. These other situations include failure of weight loss, or late regain of weight after initial success. At other times intractable GI dysfunction such as severe GERD or diarrhea may require surgical revision. Revisional surgery specifically for malnutrition is relatively rare, especially for purely restrictive procedures. For example, after LAGB, malnutrition is managed by deflation of the band, and after sleeve gastrectomy nutrition may be improved by dilation of the gastric sleeve or temporary stent insertion (Figure 8). One exception is the subset of patients who had some kind of banded gastroplasty in the past, in which case the band can be removed and the pouch of stomach used as the basis for a conventional gastric bypass. When malnutrition complicates banded GBP, as is the form of operation recommended by Fobi et al, the band is simply removed. In most cases this can be accomplished laparoscopically.

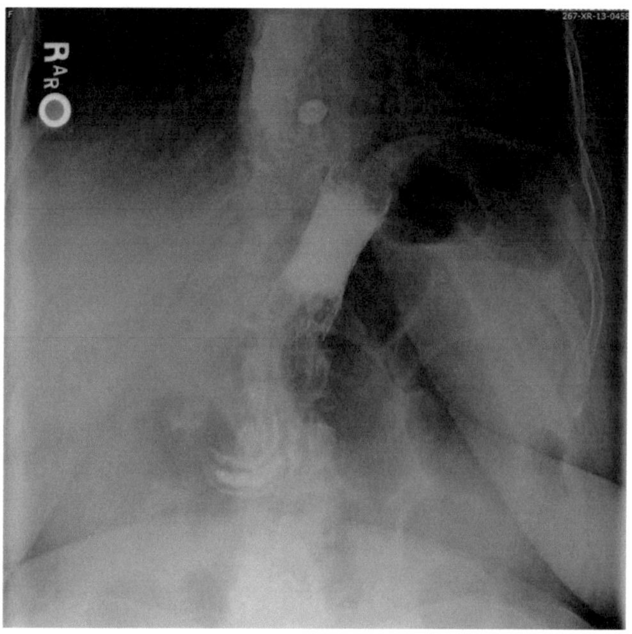

Figure 8. Correction of severe dysphagia after sleeve gastrectomy by insertion of a stent into the stomach. It is removed a few weeks later

The malabsorptive component of bariatric procedures can be reversed surgically to some extent, either by totally reversing the reconstruction or connecting the two intestinal limbs more proximally. The situation after DS is managed optimally by identifying the J-J anastomosis, and tracing the biliopancreatic and roux limbs separately, and performing a side-to-side anastomosis of the two limbs 100-200cm more proximally. This allows bile to enter the Roux limb and food to enter the biliopancreatic limb, effectively lengthening the common channel. (Figure 9) This operation, sometimes called the "Kissing X" anastomosis, effectively corrects the problems with diarrhea and hypoalbuminemia and edema [36].

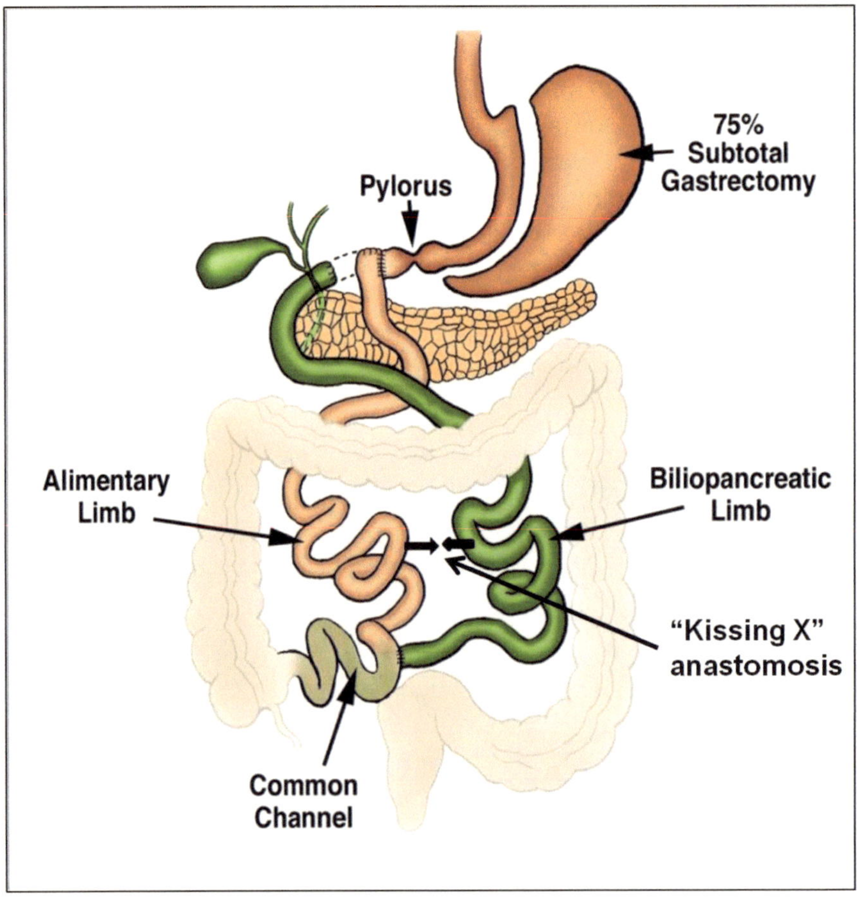

Figure 9. Correction of malabsorption by side-to-side anastomosis of the Roux limb to the Biliopancreatic limb after duodenal switch ("kissing-X" anastomosis).

In the malnourished patient after Roux Y GBP, it is simplest to insert a laparoscopic gastrostomy tube into the remnant stomach, so that all administered nutrients can be absorbed. Thereafter, the patient will be in a safer state to undergo elective reversal. Bypass reversal is accomplished by dividing the GJ anastomosis, isolating the gastric pouch, and then performing

Routine annual measurements	Purpose and clinical ituation
CBC	Basic check for anemia
CMP	Protein, liver and kidney function
Iron, TI BC, Ferritin	Adequacy of Iron stores in anemia
B12 and Folate	Work up of anemia
PTH and 25 (OH) vitamin D	Adequacy of Calcium absorption
Lipid Panel	Estimate of malabsorption
HbA1C	Monitoring diabetic resolution
Measurement in symptomatic patients	
Vitamin A	May be low in malabsorptive procedures
Vitamin B1 (whole blood)	Elucidation of neurologic or cardiac symptoms, poor oral intake or vomiting
Vitamin B6	High alcohol intake
Trace elements (Zn, Cu, Se ,Mn)	Obscure symptoms, refractory anemia especially in non-compliant patients

Table 1. List of common nutritional factors measured during routine annual follow up in patients after bariatric surgery

an anastomosis to the adjacent bypassed stomach, usually with a linear stapler. The Roux limb can simply be excised, but in a malnourished patient it is preferable to divide the original J-J anastomosis and reanastomose the limbs to restore as much intestinal absorptive area as possible.

Sometimes these operations, despite the technical simplicity, result in serious complications with catastrophic deterioration and rapid development of multi-system organ failure. The cause of such deterioration has not been established but is presumed to be due to some critical micronutrient deficiency. The most likely candidate appears to be thiamine deficiency, and anecdotal evidence has confirmed that severe hypotension with lactic acidosis may be improved by rapid administration of thiamine 100mg IV.

4.3. Specific nutritional deficiencies

4.3.1. Iron, vitamin B12 and folate

Iron deficiency is very common after any bypass operation because the maximal site of Iron absorption, the duodenum and proximal jejunum, has been bypassed. It has also been observed after sleeve gastrectomy or LAGB. Other factors contributing to Iron deficiency are the frequent use of acid suppressants, the relatively small quantities of red meat consumed by bariatric patients, and the unpleasant GI side effects associated with elemental iron ingestion. Iron deficiency is naturally commoner in menstruating women. The symptoms of anemia are so non specific – weakness, tiredness, exertional dyspnea – that measurement of routine indices is fundamental: consequently, anemia is easily and immediately recognized. Severe iron deficiency may be associated with pica, a compulsion to eat things such as crushed ice or even clay.

The treatment of iron deficiency requires replacement of iron and attention to reduce any factors exacerbating it: women with heavy menstrual losses should be referred to a gynecologist for management of menorrhagia, and acid suppression medication stopped if it is no longer necessary. Oral iron supplements are generally prescribed and include ferrous sulfate, ferrous gluconate, and ferrous fumarate. Ferrous glycine sulfate appears to have fewer side effects and the best bioavailability. Typical doses are tailored to achieve 60-100mg/day of elemental iron.

Intravenous iron supplementation may be necessary when oral iron is insufficient or cannot be tolerated. It is often administered by a hematologist in an infusion center because of concerns about allergic reactions. Intravenous iron must be complexed to other molecules to avoid iron toxicity. Iron Dextran is commonly employed. The risk of anaphylactic and other reactions is less than 1%, but recently Iron Sucrose has been used because the risk of allergic reactions is much lower (0.1%) and more recently still, Iron Carboxymaltose has been used because larger doses can be given in a short time (1000 mg over 15 minutes), making it much more convenient to administer [37].

Regardless of how iron is given, correction of anemia is a gradual process and it takes 1-2 months to restore iron and hemoglobin levels.

4.3.2. Vitamin B12 and folate

Vitamin B12 deficiency is fairly common because oral ingestion of B12 is ineffective in patients after gastric bypass, since the small gastric pouch produces so little intrinsic factor to complex with the B12 molecule. It is less likely to happen after duodenal switch or sleeve gastrectomy but it may still be present, and has been reported to be as high as 20% in some series. It typically presents a year or more after surgery because the liver has substantial reserves of B12.

Vitamin B12 deficiency causes megaloblastic anemia, which is readily correctable by restoration of B12 stores. Deficiency also predisposes to neuropsychiatric issues, causing peripheral neuropathy and symptoms of ataxia as a consequence of damage to the posterior columns of the spinal cord. There may be ataxia or inability to drive a vehicle because of loss of proprioception in the feet. These neurological symptoms may be irreversible, especially if present for longer than six months.

There is controversy about the cut-off point for the lower limit of normal for B12 levels. In USA the lower limit of normal is about 200 pg/ml, but there is concern that this level is too low and in Japan the lower limit of normal is now 550 pg/ml. In practice, it is easy to maintain healthy levels of B12 in compliant patients. Sublingual tablets permit rapid absorption without the need for intrinsic factor and are readily available over the counter in the USA. Monthly injections are also easy to administer and patients can be taught to administer such injections themselves.

Folate participates in the same pathway as vitamin B12 and is associated with similar hematologic and neurologic manifestations. It is easy to absorb and since it is a major component of multivitamin pills deficiency is rarely seen. In fact elevated levels of folate are frequently observed and generally indicate small intestinal bacterial overgrowth (SIBO).

4.3.3. Calcium and vitamin D

Calcium is another critical divalent cation which is absorbed proximally in the jejunum and may become deficient after bariatric surgery. Absorption of calcium requires vitamin D, a fat soluble sterol with many different properties. Vitamin D is initially hydroxylated in the liver to become 25 (OH) Vitamin D, and then converted to its active form, namely 1, 25 $(OH)_2$ Vitamin D in the kidney. Vitamin D is also produced by the action of UV light on the skin and in practice this is the major source of vitamin D. Vitamin D deficiency is common in northern latitudes where available sunlight exposure is limited, and also in certain ethnic subgroups where exposure of the skin to sunlight is limited for cultural reasons. Deficiency of calcium can often be detected clinically by a positive Chvostek sign, and biochemically is generally associated with elevated Parathyroid Hormone (PTH) levels.

Prolonged vitamin D deficiency causes osteomalacia, visible radiologically as loss of bone matrix, and clinically presenting with bone pain and predisposing to long bone or vertebral fractures. It also causes a proximal myopathy, especially in the muscles of the hip girdle, making it difficult to perform such simple activities as standing up from a sitting position. Typically patients rising from a chair will use their hands and arms to assist the activity, analogous to Gowers' sign observed in children with muscular dystrophy. These musculoskeletal symptoms are often dismissed as arthritis or fibromyalgia and it is important to make the diagnosis before the patient ends up being referred to a pain management clinic [38]. Vitamin D has many other advantageous qualities, including improved resistance to hospital acquired infections. [39]

Patients should have annual measurement of [25] OH Vitamin D and PTH. Low Vitamin D levels (< 30 ng/ml) require higher doses of Vitamin D than are typically present in multivitamin tablets (400 IU). The patient should have 50, 000 IU weekly and the level rechecked after 3 months. Parenteral Vitamin D is rarely required. Bone density measurements are generally within the purview of the primary care doctor, but the surgeon should regularly update and even educate the primary doctor about the patients' progress.

4.3.4. Vitamin A

Deficiency of Vitamin A is principally observed in malabsorptive operations such as DS or BPD, or the Long Limb gastric bypass. The clinical problems are chiefly ocular, and both the retina and the cornea are affected. The earliest manifestation may be night blindness, but corneal irritation and the development of Bitot's spots can also occur. There may be dry skin and dry hair and pruritus. The ocular manifestations are generally reversible when adequate supplementation is provided. The recommended dose is 10, 000 Units daily.

4.3.5. Vitamin B1

Water soluble vitamins, with the exception of vitamin B12, are not appreciably stored in the body and must be replenished regularly. Awareness amongst healthcare professionals and the lay public tends to promote the consumption of vitamin supplements and vitamin-rich foods, so that deficiency of water soluble vitamins is rarely a problem except in certain well defined groups. These include patients after bariatric surgery, alcoholics, and patients with short-gut syndromes. The importance of vitamin B12 and folate has been emphasized already. However, deficiency of vitamin B1 (Thiamine) has recently received considerable attention because it may present after periods of vomiting, such as can be frequent early after bariatric surgery of any type. A patient returning to the hospital because of intractable vomiting in the early weeks after bariatric surgery is at risk of developing thiamine deficiency. It can cause irreversible neurologic changes, with confusion, ataxia and nystagmus (Wernicke's encephalopathy) as well as heart failure [40].

Thiamine is an essential cofactor in the metabolism of glucose, and in its absence pyruvate cannot be processed in the citric acid cycle and is instead converted to lactate. The result is a serious metabolic derangement with lactic acidosis and hypotension requiring high doses of pressors. Such a patient is likely to be diagnosed with sepsis and given large volumes of fluid. Administration of dextrose in the IV fluids makes the situation worse because the glucose load cannot be metabolized. The patient should be given 200mg thiamine IV immediately and repeated daily until the patient can take a diet reliably. The cardiac failure may be rapidly improved by aggressive supplementation but the changes in Wernicke's encephalopathy may be permanent.

4.3.6. Rarer deficiencies: Vitamin B6, C, E, and trace elements

Other micronutrient deficiencies may involve other B vitamin deficiencies, but these are generally overshadowed by the major factors discussed above. Vitamins C and E have been found to be subnormal in some follow up studies after bariatric surgery. One recent report of an isolated case of severe scurvy described a patient with large confluent ecchymoses who developed multi-system organ failure, initially thought to be due to sepsis but which recovered after aggressive vitamin C replacement. Finally, there are isolated reports of trace element deficiencies, most notably Zinc, Copper and Selenium, which are important to consider in cases where unusual features of illness do not fall into a well-known pattern. Zinc deficiency appears to produce a scaly rash associated with edema. Copper deficiency produces refractory anemia and neurologic symptoms. It should always be considered in cases of refractory anemia which do not respond to iron and B12 and folate supplementation. Selenium has been implicated in a case of refractory heart failure after BPD. These micronutrients are usually a manifestation of lack of compliance since the necessary supplements are well absorbed and easy to obtain.

Taken together, these deficiencies have drawn attention to the profundity of the metabolic alteration which bariatric surgery and its altered eating behavior induces. They also emphasize the importance of facilitating long term follow up by knowledgeable providers. Prevention and management of most of these deficiencies is fairly simple when the patient remains in regular contact with the bariatric program. Regular follow up to inquire about eating habits and obtain regular laboratory monitoring of nutritional status will prevent most serious problems. Ironically, patients who are doing poorly for whatever reason may be reluctant to return to the surgeon's office because of feelings of failure or shame and thus the patients most in need of expert help are the hardest to reach. This tendency should reinforce in bariatric programs the wisdom of offering ready access and a non-judgmental attitude.

4.4. Weight regain

Weight regain after initial weight loss can be thought of as the polar opposite of malnutrition. This is the emerging as the greatest threat in the long term management of the bariatric patient. There is no clear consensus on its incidence or severity, but it is estimated that upwards of 20% of patients will regain a large proportion of the weight initially lost, and re-enter the category of morbid obesity. Why some patients do this is not known, but the causes can be thought of in two broad categories: (1) surgical factors and (2) lifestyle factors. The major surgical factors are the size of the pouch and the size of the anastomosis. Where both are small, as they are generally made these days, regain of weight is reduced. Large pouches and wider anastomoses allow greater food intake with les satiety. Sometimes the pouch is larger than the surgeon intended because a hiatal hernia was present but unrecognized.

It is widely believed, largely on anecdotal evidence that behavioral factors are the most important factors in weight regain. Patients who do not use the "honeymoon" period (the first 6-12 months when weight loss is occurring rapidly) to bring about major changes in eating and exercise patterns will gain weight in subsequent years when the restriction has worn off. Sometimes the inability to eat leads to the development of other addictions such as alcohol. Other stressful social factors, such as divorce or loss of employment, may push the patient in the direction of her old habits.

The treatment of weight regain is very problematic from many points of view. There may be no clear anatomical explanation. Patients frequently request reoperation with great fervency, not realizing that the risk of serious complications may be up to ten times greater than that of the initial surgery. If there is no identifiable mechanical reason for the weight gain, reoperation may bring about some weight loss initially, but may only set the stage for weight gain once more. Further, insurance companies frequently deny requests for authorization to perform revisional bariatric surgery for weight regain. Only if an identifiable complication such as GERD is found will the company generally authorize it. The options are either to make the pouch and anastomosis smaller, or to convert the operation to a different type of procedure [41].

If there is no clear abnormality to correct, the surgical strategy has been whimsically summarized as "bypassing the band, and banding the bypass." Patients with unsatisfactory weight loss after LAGB may be converted to RNY GBP, but the risk of leakage is higher. Failure of the RNYGBP has been reported to respond to placement of a laparoscopic band round the gastric pouch to re-impose a sense of restriction. However both these strategies are only reported in case series with limited follow up and so are only recommended on an individualized basis [42, 43].

In concert with weight regain is the recent recognition that Type 2 diabetes sometimes returns. Even when it does, it is rarely as severe as it was preoperatively. The incidence is not known but it may be as high as 30% of patients who were diabetic and who experience relief early after surgery.

4.5. Psychiatric complications

Patients who are dependent on psychiatric medications may readily suffer exacerbation of their psychiatric conditions if early swallowing and eating difficulty prevents them from resuming their normal medications. Later in the evolution of the postoperative course, they may require increasing doses (particularly antidepressants) because the reconstructed intestine absorbs less, leading to lower blood levels of the medication. For this reason many surgeons attempt to prevent such a crisis by inserting a gastrostomy tube into the remnant stomach at the time of the original bariatric procedure and remove it only when the patient is reliably consuming essential medications orally.

Some patients who have a so-called addictive personality become obese because food acts as an addictive substance and after surgery such patients may develop so-called addiction transfer, and become addicted to alcohol, drugs, or gambling.

Although most patients note enhancement of their psychosocial functioning after major weight loss, it can result in serious interpersonal conflict within families and there is a substantial incidence of breakup within marriages and domestic partnerships [44].

4.6. The disappointed patient

Some patients even without experiencing a complication may nevertheless be disappointed in the outcome, either because their weight loss was less than expected, or weight was regained a few years later, or because of the appearance of large floppy folds of skin on the abdomen, under the arms, the medial thighs and buttocks. Although these can often be dealt with by plastic surgery, such operations are themselves prone to complications of infection and seroma formation. These problems emphasize the importance of preoperative counseling and creation of realistic expectations, and the provision of postoperative counseling to assist patients in maximizing the effect of such benefits as they have achieved.

Author details

Young Kim and Peter F. Crookes*

*Address all correspondence to: peter.crookes@med.usc.edu

Department of Surgery, Keck School of Medicine, University of Southern California, Los Angeles, CA, USA

References

[1] Lancaster RT, Hutter MM. Bands and bypasses: 30-day morbidity and mortality of bariatric surgical procedures as assessed by prospective, multi-center, risk-adjusted ACS-NSQIP data. Surg Endosc 2008; 22:2554.

[2] Khan MA, Grinberg R, Johnson S, Afthinos JN, Gibbs KE. Perioperative risk factors for 30-day mortality after bariatric surgery: is functional status important? Surg Endosc 2013; 27: 1772-1777

[3] Pryor HI, Singleton A, Lin E, Lin P, Vaziri K. Practice patterns in high-risk bariatric venous thromboembolism prophylaxis. Surg Endosc 2013 27: 834-8

[4] Stein PD, Matta F. Pulmonary Embolism and deep venous thrombosis following bariatric surgery. Obes Surg 2013: 23, 663-668

[5] Sapala JA, Wood MH, Schuhknecht MP, Sapala MA. Fatal pulmonary embolism after bariatric operations for morbid obesity: a 24-year retrospective analysis. Obes Surg 2003; 13:819.

[6] Li W, Gorecki P, Semaan E, Briggs W, Tortolani AJ, D'Ayala M. Concurrent prophylactic placement of inferior vena cava filter in gastric bypass and adjustable banding operations in the Bariatric Outcomes Longitudinal Database. J Vasc Surg 2012; 55: 1690-5

[7] Becattini C, Agnelli G, Manina G, et al. Venous thromboembolism after laparoscopic bariatric surgery for morbid obesity: clinical burden and prevention. Surg Obes Relat Dis 2012; 8:108.

[8] Muorelo R, Kaidar-Person O, Fajnwaks P, Roa PE, Pinto D, Szomstein S, Rosenthal RJ Hemorrhage and thromboembolic complications after bariatric surgery in patients receiving chronic anticoagulation therapy. Obes Surg 2008; 18: 167-70

[9] Ferreira LE, Song LM, Baron TH. Management of acute postoperative hemorrhage in the bariatric patient. Gastrointest Endosc Clin N Am. 2011;21:287–294

[10] Nguyen NT, Rivers R, Wolfe BM. Early gastrointestinal hemorrhage after laparoscopic gastric bypass. Obes Surg 2003;13:62–6

[11] Bakhos C, Alkhoury F, Kyriakides T, Reinhold R, Nadzam G. Early postoperative hemorrhage after open and laparoscopic roux-en-y gastric bypass. Obes Surg 2009;19:153–157

[12] Awais O, Raftopoulos I, Luketich JD, Courcoulas A. Acute, complete proximal small bowel obstruction after laparoscopic gastric bypass due to intraluminal blood clot formation. Surg Obes Relat Dis. 2005; 4:418-22

[13] Thodiyil P, Yenumula P, Rogula T, Gorecki P, Fahoum B, Gourash W, Ramanathan R, Mattar S, Wise L, Schauer P Selective Non-operative Management of Leaks after

Gastric Bypass: Lessons Learned From 2675 Consecutive Patients. Ann Surg 2008; 248:782-792

[14] Baltasar A, Serra C, Bengochea M, Bou R, Andreo L. Use of Roux limb as remedial surgery for sleeve gastrectomy fistulas. Surg Obes Relat Dis. 2008; 4: 759-763

[15] Hii MW, ClarkeNE, HopkinsGH.Gastro-gastric herniation: an unusual complication following greater curve plication for the treatment of morbid obesity. Ann R Coll Surg Engl 2012;94:e76–8.

[16] Watkins BM. Gastric compartment syndrome: an unusual complication of gastric plication surgery. Surg Obes Relat Dis 2012;8: e80–1.

[17] Tsang A, JainV. Pitfalls of bariatric tourism: a complication of gastric plication. Surg Obes Relat Dis 2012;8:e77–9

[18] Goitein D, Matter I, Raziel A, Keidar A, Hazzan D, Rimon U, Sakran N. Portomesenteric thrombosis following laparoscopic bariatric surgery: incidence, patterns of clinical presentation, and etiology in a bariatric patient population. JAMA Surg 2013;148(4):340-6

[19] Bostanjian D, Anthone GJ, Hamoui N, Crookes PF. Rhabdomyolysis of gluteal muscles leading to renal failure: a potentially fatal complication of surgery in the morbidly obese. Obesity Surgery 2003; 13:302-5

[20] Rodriguez Uranga JJ, Ucles Sanchez AJ, Perez Diaz JM. Neuropathy of common sciatic nerve secondary to compartment syndrome as a complication after bariatric surgery. Neurologia 2005;20(2):94–7

[21] Abarbanel JM, Berginer VM, Osimani A, et al. Neurologic complications after gastric restriction surgery for morbid obesity. Neurology 1987;37(2):196–200.

[22] Thaisetthawatkul P, Collazo-Clavell ML, Sarr MG, et al. A controlled study of peripheral neuropathy after bariatric surgery. Neurology 2004;63(8):1462–70.

[23] Capella RF, Iannace VA, Capella JF. Bowel obstruction after open and laparoscopic gastric bypass surgery for morbid obesity. J Am Coll Surg 2006;203(3):328–35.

[24] Lockhart ME, Tessler FN, Canon CL, Smith JK, Larrison MC, Fineberg NS, Roy BP, Clements RH. Internal hernia after gastric bypass: Sensitivity and specificity of seven CT signs with surgical correlation and controls. Am J Roentgenol 2007; 188, 745-750

[25] Nguyen NT, Stevens CM, Wolfe BM. Incidence and outcome of anastomotic stricture after laparoscopic gastric bypass. J Gastrointest Surg 2003;7:997–1003

[26] Carter PR, LeBlanc KA, Hausmann MG, Kleinpeter KP, deBarros SN, Jones SM. Association between gastroesophageal reflux disease and laparoscopic sleeve gastrectomy. Surg Obes Rel Dis; 7: 569-572, 2012

[27] Himpens J, Dobbeleir J, Peeters G. Long-term results of laparoscopic sleeve gastrectomy for obesity. Ann Surg 2010; 252:319–324

[28] Service GJ, Thompson GB, Service FJ, Andrews JC, Collazo-Clavell ML, Lloyd RV. Hyperinsulinemic hypoglycemia with nesidioblastosis after gastric bypass surgery N Engl J Med. 2005;353(3):249-54

[29] Mala T. Postprandial Hyperinsulinemic hypoglycemia after gastric bypass surgical treatment. Surg Obes Rel Dis; 2014 (epub ahead of print)

[30] Lazzati A, Polliand C, Porta M, Torcivia A, Paolino LA, Champault G, Barrat C. Is fixation during gastric banding necessary? A randomized clinical study. Obes Surg 2011;21:1859-63

[31] Brown WA, Egberts KJ, Franke-Richard D, Thodiyil P, Anderson ML, O'Brien PE. Erosions after adjustable gastric banding: diagnosis and management. Ann Surg (2013); 257:1047-1052

[32] El-Hayek K, Timratana P, Brethauer SA, Chand B. Complete endoscopic/transgastric retrieval of eroded gastric band: description of a novel technique and review of the literature. Surg Endosc 2013; 27(8):2974-9

[33] Ziegler O, Sirveaux MA, Brunaud L, Reibel N, Quilliot D. Medical follow up after bariatric surgery: nutritional and drug issues. General recommendations for the prevention and treatment of nutritional deficiencies. Diabet Metab. 2009;35:544–557

[34] Fujioka K. Follow-up of nutritional and metabolic problems after bariatric surgery. Diabetes Care 2005;28:481–484

[35] Gasteyger C, Suter M, Gaillard RC, Giusti V Nutritional deficiencies after Roux-en-Y gastric bypass for morbid obesity often cannot be prevented by standard multivitamin supplementation. Am J Clin Nutr. 2008; 87:1128-33

[36] Hamoui N, Chock B, Anthone GJ, Crookes PF. Revision of the duodenal switch: indications, technique, and outcomes. J Am Coll Surg 2007;204:603-8.

[37] Lyseng-Williamson KA, Keating GM. Ferric carboxymaltose: a review of its use in iron-deficiency anaemia. Drugs. 2009; 69:739-56.

[38] Girgis CM, Clifton-Bligh RJ, Hamrick MW, Holick MF, Gunton JE. The roles of vitamin D in skeletal muscle: form, function, and metabolism. Endocr Rev. 2013;34:33-83.

[39] Quraishi SA, Bittner EA, Blum L, Hutter MM, Camargo CA Jr. Association between preoperative 25-hydroxyvitamin D level and hospital-acquired infections following Roux-en-Y gastric bypass surgery. JAMA Surg 2014;149:112-8

[40] Milone M, Di Minno MN, Lupoli R, Maietta P, Bianco P, Pisapia A, Gaudioso D, Taffuri C, Milone F, Musella M. Wernicke encephalopathy in subjects undergoing restrictive weight loss surgery: a systematic review of literature data. Eur Eat Disord Rev. 2014;22:223-9

[41] Shimizu H, Annaberdyev S, Motamarry I, Kroh M, Schauer PR, Brethauer SA Revisional bariatric surgery for unsuccessful weight loss and complications. Obes Surg 2013;23:1766-73

[42] Irani K, Youn HA, Ren-Fielding CJ, Fielding GA. Midterm results for gastric banding as salvage procedure for patients with weight loss failure after Roux-en-Y gastric bypass. Surg Obes Relat Dis. 2011;7:219-2

[43] Brown JJ, Boyle M, Mahawar K, Balupuri S, Small PK. Laparoscopic adjustable gastric band survival in a high-volume bariatric unit. Br J Surg 2013; 100:1614-8

[44] Rand CSW, Juldau JM, Robbins L. Surgery for obesity and marriage quality. JAMA 1982;247: 1419–1422.

Section 2

New Bariatric Surgery and Indication

Chapter 4

Bariatric Surgery in Adolesencets : a multidisciplinary Approach

Yu JIanchun

Additional information is available at the end of the chapter

http://dx.doi.org/10.5772/58624

1. Introduction

Great societal changes have be found in the world with fast lifestyle, less activity or exercises in recent 30 years. The epidemic of obesity continues to grow and affect almost every aspect of the lives of patients and human life especially in children and adolencents. The growing prevalence of diabetes and cardiovascular disease (CVD) parallels the increased revalence of obesity.

The Center for Disease Control (CDC) in the United States defines overweight as a body mass index(BMI, kg/m^2) of 25.0 to 29.9 and obesity as a BMI greater than 30.0 kg/m^2. It is different from CDC in Asia or in China with the definition as overweight 24.0 to 27.9 and obesity as a BMI greater than 28.0 kg/m^2.

Obesity is strongly associated with severe medical problems including increased risk for cardiovascular morbidity and mortality, hypertension, cholethiasis, nonalcoholic steatohepatitis (NASH), sleep apnea, orthopedic dysfunction, depression, breast, colon and uterine cancers. The disease profile changes in the adolencent population increasing of metabolic syndrome or Type II diabetes and cancer. The great challenges associated with or directly responsible for multiple medical problems or comorbidities to the traditional culture, education, medical system, multidisciplinary medical workers and healthy professionals.

It necessitates attention to care bariatric healthcare professionals. A multidisciplinary Approach, to help healthcare professionals navigate the difficult road of treating adolescent obesity.

INTECH
open science | open minds

© 2014 The Author(s). Licensee InTech. This chapter is distributed under the terms of the Creative Commons Attribution License (http://creativecommons.org/licenses/by/3.0), which permits unrestricted use, distribution, and reproduction in any medium, provided the original work is properly cited.

2. The causes of obesity

The causes of obesity are multifactorial roles with genetics, environmental factors, food consumption, and family interactions.

All obese children and adults develop from consistaining a positive-balance between energy intake (high-calorie, nutrient-dense foods) and energy output (physical activity and exercise). Parents have a major influence on their children regarding their intake and activity/inactivity. Children from overweight/obese families have higher obesity rate with low cognitive stimulation and less physical activity than normal weight families

Exercise Prescription Guidelines for the obese Child and Adolecents

The emergence of Type 2 diabetes (T2D) in children and adolescents parallels the rising rates of childhood obesity. As a condition of impaired insulin sensitivity and relative insulin deficiency resulting in hyperglycemia, T2D has a complex underlying physiology that is reflected by the multiple approaches used to optimize medical care and prevent the myriad of diabetes-related complications [2].

Chinese famous philosopher Lao-Tzu said: The journey of a thousand miles begins with the first step.

All the children and adolescents need eating disorder treatment [3]. They need an negative-balance between energy intake (low-calorie, nutrient-dense foods) and energy output (physical activity and exercise). Obese children or adolences have to work harder than normal weight children or adolences to accomplish the same task and thus need adjusted workloads. An exercise program and assessment for obese child and adolescents should be designed to increase caloric expenditure rather than to improve cardiovascular fitness. However, medical intervention is failure for long-term weight loss in most morbidly obese persons.

3. Effect of weight reduction or bariatric surgery in type 2 diabetes and prediabetes

It has been demonstrated that weight reduction – even modest loss of 6 to 10 percent had a remarkable effect on diabetes control in patients with type 2 diabetes and reduced the risk for prediatetes patient developing to diabetes by a profound effect on preventing natural progression of glucose intolerance from IGT to type 2 diatetes.

The weight reduction reduces the incidence of most obesity complications and improves overall sense of wellbeing. Although lifestyle modification has been the traditional clinical recommendation for overweightand obese prediabetic and diabetic patients, bariatric surgery became another valid and effective option for long-term weight control among these high risk patients because diabetes is a major comorbid condition.

The incidence of adolescent bariatric surgery is increasing with safely as evidenced by low complication rates [5]. Extremely obese diabetic adolescents experience significant weight loss and remission of type 2 diabetes mellitus after Roux-en-Y gastric bypass with Improvements in insulin resistance, beta-cell function, and cardiovascular risk factors support Roux-en-Y gastric bypass as an intervention that improves the health of these adolescents. It suggests that Roux-en-Y gastric bypass is an effective option for the treatment of extremely obese adolescents with type 2 diabetes mellitus [6].

4. Indications for bariatric surgery

The 1998 NHLBI obesity clinical guidelines for adults set the patient selection criterion for obesity surgery as a BMI of 40 or more or a BMI between 35 and 40 accompanied by high-risk obesity cormobidities such as type 2 diatetes, hypertension, sleep apnea, asthma, or osteoarthritis of weight-bearing joints. Surgery is recommended only for patients who have an acceptable risk for surgery, are well-informed, motivated, and able to participate in treatment and long-term follow-up. Patients who choose surgery will require lifelong medical care and should work with a multidisplinary team including medical, nutritional, and behavioral specialists (NHLBI, 1998). While the NIH guidelines have remained unchanged since 1991. Newer criteria for adults are being evaluated. The current BMI standard is changed by evidence that bariatric surgery can reverse comorbidities such as type 2 diabetes even in patients with a BMI of less than 30 (Pories, 2010) or 28 (Huang ZK,) that applying an adjusted BMI which takes into account race, sex, age, fitness, or body fat composition, would be a more realistic criterion.

5. Opinions of healthcare professionals in the world regarding bariatric surgery

Opinions of healthcare professionals in the world regarding bariatric surgery in adolescents are largely unknown. Although surgery may be a promising treatment for extreme obesity in youth, the acceptability of bariatric surgical interventions for obese children and adolescents remains a topic of controversy among patients, healthcare practitioners, researchers, policy-makers, and general public. An investigation study on the disagreement of bariatric surgery for adolescent showed that almost half of the participating physicians would never refer an obese adolencent for a bariatric operation, some physicians would referred with the minimum age of 18 years (Woolford, 2010).

There is a study from the UK to explore the perspectives of medical professionals regarding adolescent bariatric surgery [7]. Members of the British Obesity and Metabolic Surgery Society and groups of primary care practitioners based in London were contacted by electronic mail and invited to complete an anonymous online survey consisting of 21 questions. 66% of professionals felt that adolescents with a body mass index (BMI) >40 or BMI >35 with significant co-morbidities can be offered surgery. Amongst pre-requisites, parental psychological counseling was chosen most frequently. 58% stated 12 months as an appropriate period for weight management programs, with 24% regarding 6 months as sufficient. Most participants believed bariatric surgery should only be offered ≥16 years of age. However, 17% of bariatric surgeons marked no minimum age limit. Over 80% of the healthcare professionals surveyed consider bariatric surgery in adolescents to be acceptable practice. Most healthcare professionals surveyed feel that adolescent bariatric surgery is an acceptable therapeutic option for adolescent obesity. These views can guide towards a consensus opinion and further development of selection criteria and care pathways.

6. Age limits

There are some specific limit for bariatric surgery although it may achieve a sustained weight loss. For old adults age guidelines from the American Society for Metabolic & Bariatric Surgery (ASMES) suggest that patients eligible for surgery should be 18 to 65 years old. Individuals outside that age range who undergo surgery should have significant health conditions related to obesity and the expectation of improved life expectancy or quality of life should outweigh the risk of surgery (Mechanick, 2008). The NHLBI clinical guidelines summarized the available data regarding any type of weight reduction after age 65 and recommended: A clinical decision to forgo obesity treatment in an older adult should be guided by an evaluation of the potential benefits of weight reduction for day-to –day functioning and reduction of the risk of future cardiovascular events, as well as the patient's motivation for weight reduction. (NHLBI, 1998).

The recommendations are supported by the Pediatric Surgical Association and the American Society of Bariatric Surgery based on the opinions of "experts". The adolescents should be limited in age for girls (13 years) and boys (15 years).

6.1. Contraindication

The suggested contraindications would include an extremly high operative risk, such as severe cardiovascular disease or severe respiratory problems. To help avoid adverse postoperative outcomes, patients are also screened for sevsere depression, untreated mental illnesses, active substance abuse, or binge eating disorders, severe cardiovascular disease or severe respiratory problems. Patients who cannot comprehend the nature of the surgical intervention and the lifelong measures required to maintain health, should not be offered this procedure (Mechanick, 2008).

7. Surgery for severe obesity

Although the increasing incidence of obesity is due to an imbalance of energy intake and energe output, long-term weight loss is difficult to achive with diet, exercise, or pharmacotherapy. Lack effective treatment for obesity is also a significant contributor to this serious public health problem. To date, bariatric surgery has been shown to be the only intervention to induce significant weight loss in patients with severe obesity and improve chronic health conditions, survival, and quality of life. Most bariatric surgery patients have already experienced numerous attempts to achieve a sustained weight loss by using nonsurgical treatment options.

Bariatric surgical procedures have increased exponentially for Severe Obesity in the world. The three commonly performed procedures in obeses aldults are laparoscopic Roux-en-Y gastric bypass (LRYGB), laparoscopic adjustable gastric banding (LAGB), and the novel laparoscopic sleeve gastrectomy (LSG) have acceptable efficacy and safety for resolution of obesity-related comorbidities [8] The best option from the different developing surgery procedures with evaluated results are the new clinical problems.

A systematic literature review (2004 from Royal Australasian College of Surgeons) compare the safety and efficacy of laparoscopic adjustable gastric banding with vertical-banded gastroplasty and gastric bypass [9]. The results showed that LAGB was associated with a mean short-term mortality rate of approximately 0.05% and an overall median morbidity rate of approximately 11.3%, compared with 0.50% and 23.6% for RYGB, and 0.31% and 25.7% for VBG. Overall, all 3 procedures produced considerable weight loss in patients up to 4 years in the case of LAGB (the maximum follow-up available at the time of the review), and more than 10 years in the case of the comparator procedures. The Australian Safety and Efficacy Register of New Interventional Procedures-Surgical Review Group concluded that the evidence base was of average quality up to 4 years for LAGB. Laparoscopic gastric banding is safer than VBG and RYGB, in terms of short-term mortality rates. LAGB is effective, at least up to 4 years, as are the comparator procedures. Up to 2 years, LAGB results in less weight loss than RYGB; from 2 to 4 years there is no significant difference between LAGB and RYGB, but the quality of data is only moderate. Although Laparoscopic adjustable gastric banding is now promoted as a safer, potentially reversible and effective alternative to Roux-en-Y gastric bypass.

A systematic review [10] comparing the two most popular bariatric procedures-Gastric banding or bypass? The conclusion strongly favored Roux-en-Y gastric bypass over laparoscopic adjustable gastric banding for weight loss outcomes. Patients treated with laparoscopic adjustable gastric banding had lower short-term morbidity than those treated with Roux-en-Y gastric bypass, but reoperation rates were higher among patients who received laparoscopic adjustable gastric banding. Gastric bypass should remain the primary bariatric procedure used to treat obesity in the United States. Lee WJ [11] conducted a randomized trial of moderately obese Chinese patients (BMI < 35) with troublesome, difficult diabetes. Patients were followed for 1 year. Nearly all patients (93%) in the gastric bypass group had a remission of diabetes, compared with less than half of patients (47%) with sleeve gastrectomy. Weight loss was also more pronounced after gastric bypass. A meta-analysis of international bariatric surgery studies from 2003 to 2012 provides reassurance that the surgery is effective for candidates of procedures with 3 main types of bariatric surgery [12]. Gastric bypass resulted in more effective weight loss, but was associated with more complications. Adjustable gastric banding was linked with lower mortality and complication rates; however, it had a higher reoperation rate and was associated with less substantial weight loss than gastric bypass. Sleeve gastrectomy, which is becoming more popular, resulted in weight loss comparable to that obtained with gastric bypass and greater than that with adjustable.

A first report [13] from the American College of Surgeons Bariatric Surgery Center Network showed showed that laparoscopic sleeve gastrectomy has morbidity and effectiveness positioned between the band and the bypass. for data up to 1 year.

A retrospective short-and mid-term follow-up of a single institution of the American College of Surgeons Bariatric Surgery Centers of Excellence reviewed the experience and the procedure-related morbidity among all 3 procedures between the years 2005 and 2011 to identified and compared complications, mortality, readmissions, and reoperations in patients who underwent LRYGB, LAGB, and LSG. A total of 2,199 bariatric procedures were performed during this period of time. Of those procedures, 1,327 were LRYGB, 619 were LSG, and 253 were LAGB. Perioperative mortality was not applicable for all 3 procedures. The leak rate was 0.5% for LRYGB and 0.3% for LSG, and was not applicable for LAGB. The average number of readmissions postoperatively was less than 2 times for all 3 procedures: LRYGB 1.96 times, LSG 1.49 times, and LAGB 1.54 times. The percentages of procedures requiring reoperations due to complications or failures were 14.6% in the LAGB group, 6.6% in the LRYGB group, and 1.8% in the LSG group. The conclusion showed that LSG appears to have the lowest procedure-related morbidity when compared with LRYGB and LAGB in short-and mid-term follow-up [14].

8. Bariatric surgery in adolescents

Medical therapy to lose weight including exercise, diet, psychological behavior modification, and pharmacotherapy. Published long-term in obese and morbidly obese patients are non-existent. It is estimated that failure of medical therapy to reduce significant weight for a sustained a mount of time is close to 100 percent in the morbidly obese person.

Surgery as an alternative procedure to treat morbidly obese patients was first performed in the mil-1960s with the negative results due to high incidence of complications, temporary weight loss, and significant metabolic complications. In the last decade, the laparoscopic minimally invasive procedures performed to treat morbid obesity have been established as preferred weight loss method for safe and effectiveness with 20 years follow-up with less comorbidities.

An increasing number of young people with a BMI of greater than 40 and severe comorbidities, such as type 2 diatetes, and sleep apnea, are undergonging bariatric surgery. Supporting research shows bariatric surgery in adolescents is associated with weight loss, reducing the risks associated with metabolic disorders, and improved self-image and socialization (Lawson, 2006; Xanthakos, 2008). Long-term data including information on malabsorption of critical nutrients and effects on maturation is needed by long-term follow-up MDT clinical study. Experts advise that bariatric surgical therapy should be reserved for full-grow adolescents with treatment by experienced multidisciplinary teams who can provide comprehensive medical and psychological care (Livingston, 2010b). Bariatric procedures are generally contraindicated for preadolescent age groups, as long-term health effects, durability of the weight loss, and life expectancy for teens who undergo operations remain largely unknown.

The lack of data regarding bariatric surgery in adolescents has created a significant controversy regarding the benefits and indications.

Bariatric surgery should be offered to adolescents using a set of more conservative criteria. These could include failure of medical therapy for at least 3-6 months.

Bariatric surgery is an increasingly utilized option for the treatment of morbid obesity among adolescents [15]. The procedures can be performed safely as evidenced by low complication rates. There is plenty of evidence that three procedures have been performed with LAGB, Sleeve gastrectomy and gastric bypass by the different weight loss results. The follow-up studies in 2003 showed the majority of adolescent patients with good results by losing over 50 percent of excess body weight (EBW) after LAP-BAND at 2 to 3 years and lose more weight (60-80% of EBW) after gastric bypass at 1 to 2 years.

There are very few complications with band slippage in 5 percent, port leak in 5 percent, and erosion of the band in 2 percent. Intolerance to food, nausea, and vomiting, bowel obstruction, and vitamin deficiencies or regaining problems during long-term follow-up which increased the re-operating procedures. The complications were more frequent in the gastric bypass procedure that including pulmonary embolism, strictures, anastomotic leaks and bleeding, and bowel obstructions. There are more data indicating that LAGB procedure may not be as effective in "superobese" patients (BMI > 50) because of insufficient weight loss. However, this concept is currently chanllenged by different mechanism studies in different bariatric procedures. In fact, many patients and also surgeons are preferred one procedure.

There is increasing consensus that bariatric surgery is superior to medical intervention for long-term weight loss in morbidly obese persons. Most postoperative patients are able to lose a significant amount of weight, profit from reduced or resolved comorbidities with an improved quality of life (QOL). Despite these benefits from bariatric surgery, 5-30% patients either lose little weight or unable to maintain their weight lose or regaining weight over the long term. Aside from medical or surgical complications, postoperative weight loss success depongs upon the patient's abilities and willingness with family to follow the prescribed nutritional and lifestyle guidelines by Multidisciplinary team (MDT). Whereas the surgery provides the tool for weight loss the patient must provide the motivation and ability to obtain the long-term success. New researches, mechanisms new operating options and evaluation or effects of obesity on the causes, continues to evolve.

9. Multidisciplinary care for obese patients

Obesity is strongly associated with severe medical problems. Before bariatric surgery, we need to set up the multidisciplinary team in hospital.

Multidisciplinary care for obese patient is an integrated, collaborative approach to treatment planning and ongoing patient care and management. To understand the roles and the management of MDT is important to realize the safe and effeciency for bariatric surgery purpose.

To understand the benefits of the MDT approach on obese patient outcomes, we need to know the problems of obese patients. Morbidly obese patients may have significant sympotoms of depression, evidence of eating disorders, negative body image, low QOL, and other coexisting mental disorders. Bariatric surgery candidates have a varity of psychiatric and behavioral problems such as anxiety depression, eating disorders, and history of sexual abuse. Psychopathology and various psychological difficulties exist prior to the bariatric surgery can direct adverse effects on the postoperative outcome.

Physical system exam, preoperative weight loss, psychological and preoperative tests or assessment may prove identified and valuble factors predicting postoperative success.

An MDT comprises all relevant medical and allied HCPs from different disciplines who are required to effectively plan personalised treatment and care for obese patients [17]. This involves: 1. To comprehensive review of clinical and diagnostic findings; 2. To consideration of all treatment options relevant to the case; 3. To educate the patient with the parents and families; 4. To development of an individual treatment plan for each patient. To follow-up and resolve the problems and complications such as regaining or nutrition deficiency.

The carrer of treatment for obese and morbidly obese individuals must be a multidisciplinary approach.

Members of an bariatric surgery with MDT include core members and supported members. Core members including general surgical surgeons or GI surgeons, endocrinologists, dietitians, radiaologists, cardiovascular specialists, respiratory and anesthesia specialists, psychologists and behavioral specialists. Supported members include nurses, data managers, researchers, healthcare practionares, social workers.

10. Before surgery — Psychological test and education assessment

From a psychological perspective, bariatric surgery is unique because it is a behavioral surgery in which the "outcomes are independent of the technical performance of the operation." Surgery outcome, especially long-term maintaince of weight loss, relies almost completely on patient ability and / or willingness to make significant changes in eating and exercise habits and often in the emotional relationship with food. Bariatric surgery provides anatomical tools that make it easier to restrict food consumption and nutrient absorption, allowing patients to correct imbalances in caloric intake and metabolic demand. In addition to the numerous behavioral demands following surgery, there are significant risks for serious postoperative complications, even death.

For these reasons, patient education and knowledge play critical roles in bariatric surgery, influencing nearly every part of the surgery process and outcome, including patients' abilities to give informed consent, develop realistic expectations, prepare psychologically, and succeed in making the behavioral changes that lead to sustained weight loss. Unfortuneately, there is often a gap in patient's knowledge and misconceptions about surgery that interfere with the goals. The knowledge of patient with their parents and family would impact on bariatric surgery outcome.

In order to improve the patient education process in bariatric surgery, it is necessary to identify areas of knowledge that tend to be ploblematic. It also suggested that patient knowledge needs to be assessed after educational interventions to insure that information has been assimilated.

As healthcare professionals we need continue to educate and update ourselves with the growing and difficulty road of surgical Intervention or treating obesity, weight management, and multidisciplinary approaches surrounding this obese patients with their parents and family.

11. Conclusions and recommendations

Obesity is a major worldwide problem in public health, reaching epidemic proportions in many countries, especially in urbanized regions. Bariatric procedures have been shown to be more effective in the management of morbid obesity, compared to medical treatments in terms of weight loss and its sustainability

Management of Pediatric and Adolescent Type 2 Diabetes is a special long-term healthcare and research work. All of the bariatric surgery adolescent patients should be managed in a comprehensive multidisciplinary program and operaed on in hospitals and centers with extensive experience performing bariatric surgery [16-17]. The decision and the type of surgery should be individualized for each patients and experience of the individual surgeon.

The LAGB insertion should be the first choice for adolescent patients to bring behavior changes with less obstacles to the growth after bariatric surgery. However, in recent years surgeons are likely to perform LAP-sleeve gastrectomy with the better results and less complications especially for "superobese" patients or LAGB failed patients. All the adolescent patients and their parents should be informed in detail on the advantages and disadvantages of each available procedure, possibly in several interviews and always accompanied by a specialized interdisciplinary team. The long-term follow-up evaluation. Studies should to be continued.

Author details

Yu JIanchun

GI surgery and Metabolic Nutrition Division, Dept. of general surgery, Peking Union Medical College Hospital, Chinese Academy of Medical Sciences, Beijing, China

References

[1] Alexandra G. Kazaks, Judith S. Stern. Nutrition and Obesity. Copyright © 2013 by Jones & Bartlett Learning, LLC, an Ascend Learning Company.

[2] Amed S, Daneman D, Mahmud FH, et al. Type 2 diabetes in children and adolescents. Expert Rev Cardiovasc Ther. 2010 Mar;8(3):393-406.

[3] Walker T, Watson HJ, Leach DJ, et al. Comparative study of children and adolescents referred for eating disorder treatment at a specialist tertiary setting. Int J Eat Disord. 2014 Jan;47(1):47-53.

[4] Wiegand S, Maikowski U, Blankenstein O, et al. Type 2 diabetes and impaired glucose tolerance in European children and adolescents with obesity--a problem that is no longer restricted to minority groups. Eur J Endocrinol. 2004 Aug;151(2):199-206.

[5] Zwintscher NP, Azarow KS, Horton JD, et al, The increasing incidence of adolescent bariatric surgery. J Pediatr Surg. 2013 Dec;48(12):2401-7.

[6] Inge TH, Miyano G, Bean J, et al, Reversal of type 2 diabetes mellitus and improvements in cardiovascular risk factors after surgical weight loss in adolescents. Pediatrics. 2009 Jan;123(1):214-22.

[7] Penna M, Markar S, Hewes J, et al. Adolescent Bariatric Surgery-Thoughts and Perspectives.Int J Environ Res Public Health. 2013 Dec 31;11(1):573-82.

[8] Franco JV, Ruiz PA, Palermo M, et al. A review of studies comparing three laparoscopic procedures in bariatric surgery: sleeve gastrectomy, Roux-en-Y gastric bypass and adjustable gastric banding. Obes Surg. 2011 Sep;21(9):1458-68.

[9] Chapman AE, Kiroff G, Game P, et al. Laparoscopic adjustable gastric banding in the treatment of obesity: a systematic literature review. Surgery. 2004 Mar;135(3):326-51.

[10] Tice JA, Karliner L, Walsh J, et al. Gastric banding or bypass? A systematic review comparing the two most popular bariatric procedures. Am J Med. 2008 Oct;121(10): 885-93.

[11] Lee WJ, Chong K, Ser KH, et al. Gastric bypass vs sleeve gastrectomy for type 2 diabetes mellitus: a randomized controlled trial. Arch Surg, 2011, 146(2):143-148

[12] Marlene Busko Current Bariatric Surgery Safe and Effective: Meta-analysis

[13] *JAMA Surgery* December 18, 2013 ; Medscape Medical News December 24, 2013

[14] Hutter MM, Schirmer BD, Jones DB,et al. First report from the American College of Surgeons Bariatric Surgery Center Network: laparoscopic sleeve gastrectomy has morbidity and effectiveness positioned between the band and the bypass. Ann Surg. 2011 Sep;254(3):410-20

[15] Fridman A, Moon R, Cozacov Y, et al. Procedure-related morbidity in bariatric surgery: a retrospective short-and mid-term follow-up of a single institution of the

American College of Surgeons Bariatric Surgery Centers of Excellence. J Am Coll Surg. 2013 Oct;217(4):614-20.

[16] Zwintscher NP, Azarow KS, Horton JD, et al. The increasing incidence of adolescent bariatric surgery. J Pediatr Surg. 2013 Dec;48(12):2401-7.

[17] Yu Jianchun Bariatric surgery and multidisciplinary treatment for obesity. Acta Acad Med Sin 2001, 33(3):219-223

[18] Raul J. Rosenthal, Daniel B. Jones. Weight Loss Surgery: A multidisciplinary Approach. Copyright © 2008 Matrix Medical Communications Edgemont, Pennsylvania, USA.

Chapter 5

A New Emerging procedure — Sleeve Gastrectomy

Asim Shabbir and Jun Liang Teh

Additional information is available at the end of the chapter

http://dx.doi.org/10.5772/58844

1. Introduction

Laparoscopic Sleeve Gastrectomy (LSG) is an increasingly popular procedure for weight loss. Compared to other bariatric procedures, sleeve gastrectomy remains a relatively young stand-alone weight loss operation. However, despite being relatively new it has gained grounds not only in the west where bariatric surgery has been around for long but also in Asia where it is increasingly becoming the procedure of choice for weight loss [1, 2]. Its attractiveness is attributed not only to its significant weight loss outcome, but also the technical austerity of the operation as well as the significant improvement or remission of medical co morbidities.

1.1. History

Sleeve gastrectomy may be seen as an extension of the Magenstrasse and Mill procedure. The first open sleeve gastrectomy was performed in March 1998 by Doug Hess [3]. A year later, the first laparoscopic duodenal switch with a sleeve gastrectomy was reported on a porcine model [4]. LSG was first performed in 2000, by Gagner et al as part of a duodenal switch procedure and he subsequently also reported sleeve gastrectomy after BPD/DS as a salvage procedure for poor weight loss [5, 6]. Regan et al. then reported sleeve gastrectomy as a first step for sufficient weight loss prior to performing a more definite procedure such as Roux-en-Y bypass or duodenal switch in high-risk obese patients to decrease mortality and morbidity [7].

1.2. Indications

The NIH Consensus conference [8] in 1991 stipulated that patients with BMI equal to or exceeding 40kg/m^2 or patients with high risk co-morbid conditions and BMI exceeding or equal to 35 kg/m^2 were candidates for bariatric surgery. For Asian patients, the BMI cut-off is 2.5kg/m^2 lower [9]. More recently, the International Sleeve Gastrectomy Expert

INTECH
open science | open minds

© 2014 The Author(s). Licensee InTech. This chapter is distributed under the terms of the Creative Commons Attribution License (http://creativecommons.org/licenses/by/3.0), which permits unrestricted use, distribution, and reproduction in any medium, provided the original work is properly cited.

Consensus Statement stipulated that laparoscopic sleeve gastrectomy (LSG) was a valid stand-alone procedure for patients with metabolic syndrome as well as patients with a BMI of 30 – 35 kg/m^2 in presence of associated comorbidities [10]. Obese patients with Child's A or B liver cirrhosis, inflammatory bowel disease or potential transplant recipients were also potential candidates for LSG [10]. LSG was also deemed suitable for morbidly obese patients in their adolescence as well as elderly morbidly obese patients. Medical tourism is on the rise and people traveling from far-fetched regions with minimal support may seek bariatric surgery and once stationed back in their remote locations may not have access to care needed for maintenance. A very low of long term complications is seen as an advantage to recommend this procedure.

1.3. Contraindications

LSG has been reported to increase the incidence of gastroesophageal reflux disease (GERD) [11]. A history of GERD is a relative contraindication for undergoing laparoscopic sleeve gastrectomy as their symptoms might worsen after surgery and these patients may be better served with other procedures e.g. gastric bypass [12].

Caution should be exercised in patients with concurrent Barrett's Esophagus. Performing a sleeve gastrectomy will decrease the amount of gastric tissue available for creation of a gastric tube after esophagectomy if there is malignant progression of the Barrett's Esophagus. LSG is preferred and favored over Roux-en-Y bypass in patients / regions at high risk of developing gastric cancer as performing the latter procedure will make endoscopic surveillance of the remnant stomach for cancer almost impossible.

2. The procedure

2.1. Preoperative considerations

The preoperative management does not differ from other bariatric procedures. Patients with a history of smoking should be encouraged to stop smoking. Dietary counseling should be mandatory and should address preoperative weight loss, immediate and long term diet recommendations after sleeve gastrectomy. Initiation of a low calorie diet prior to surgery should be considered as this helps shrink the large fatty liver and thus optimizes intra-abdominal operating space. Investigations to evaluate peri-operative risk, exclude other causes of obesity and those on long term follow up nutritional monitoring are a norm. A visit to a physiotherapist, psychologist, pulmonologist, anesthetist and other physicians should be considered on need basis. The role of a multidisciplinary team to manage these patients cannot be further emphasized [13].

2.2. Technique

a. Positioning

It should be ensured that the operating table has the capacity to support the weight of the patient. The patient may be positioned supine or in French position with legs apart (Figure

1). The feet are secured to the foot board so that reverse trendeleburg position is possible. The arms should be well padded to prevent neurological injury should the arms be stretched out and secured to an arm board. Once the patient is strapped down, the table should be tilted to extremes to ensure that the patient is well secured and would not slip off the table (Figure 2).

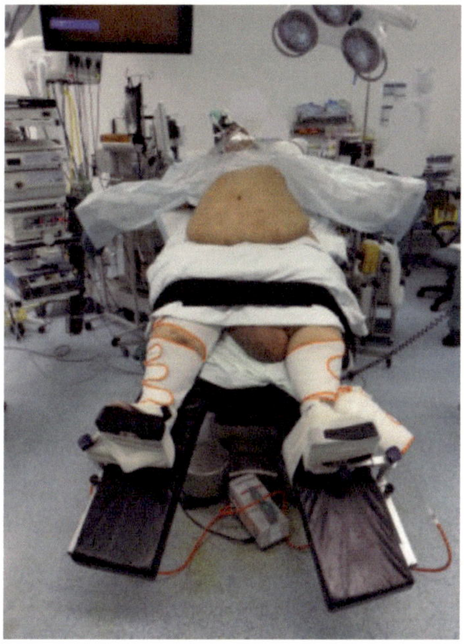

Figure 1. French position

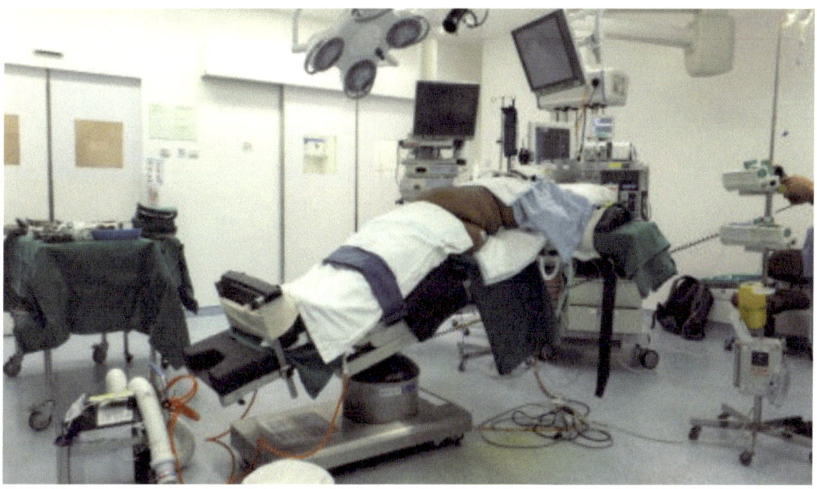

Figure 2. Patient secured on operating table

b. Decompression of the stomach

This can be achieved by insertion of orogastric tube, a hollow calibration tube by gastroscopy. We insert our disposable 38F calibration tube after positioning the patient and prior to draping. In doing so, we are able to empty the gastric contents prior to surgery and during surgery, to maneuver the calibration tube to size the sleeve. The insertion of a calibration tube is not without problems. If one faces resistance during insertion of it is better to use a gastroscope or colonoscope as calibration tube. There are reports of esophageal perforation resulting from improper handling of calibration tubes [14].

c. Port placement

5 ports are typically inserted for LSG in our patients. A 10-12 optical trocar is inserted 20 cm below the left costal margin along the midclavicular line to gain access to the abdominal cavity. Other techniques like the use of Veress needle and open Hassan technique may be used. A 5mm epigastric port is inserted for introduction of a liver retractor. For patients where the distance between the xyphoid and umbilicus is up to 35cm we insert an infra-umbilical 15mm port as the working port for the surgeon. If the distance is more or the patient has central obesity this port is changed to a 10-12mm port that is placed approximately 20cm from xyphoid to the left of the mid line. Two 5mm ports are inserted in the left and right hypochondria regions of the patient for assistant and surgeon (Figure 3).

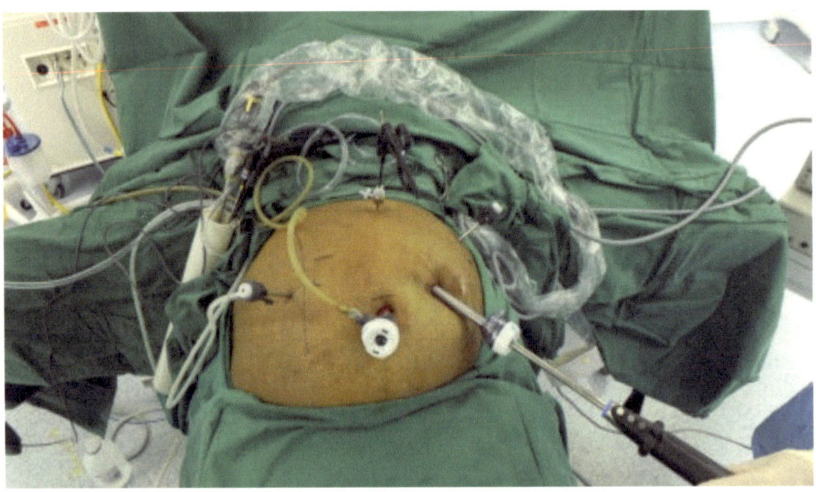

Figure 3. Port placement

d. Measurement of the Antral pouch:

Once pneumoperitoneum is established, a diagnostic laparoscopy is performed and hepatic steatosis assessed. The greater gastrocolic omentum is divided 5 cm from the pylorus with the aid of an energy device (Figure 4). There is consensus among bariatric surgeons that the antral pouch should be measured 2-6cm from the pylorus along greater curve [10] as risk benefit ratio is best within these limits. However, some surgeons also believe that cutting too close to pylorus increases risk of leak and most would prefer to stay 4-6cm away. Michalsky D et al compared patients who underwent radical resection of antrum (resection 2.5cm from pylorus) versus those with preserved antrum (resection 6cm from pylorus), they found no difference in % excess weight loss, complications, gastric emptying and food retention between both groups [15].

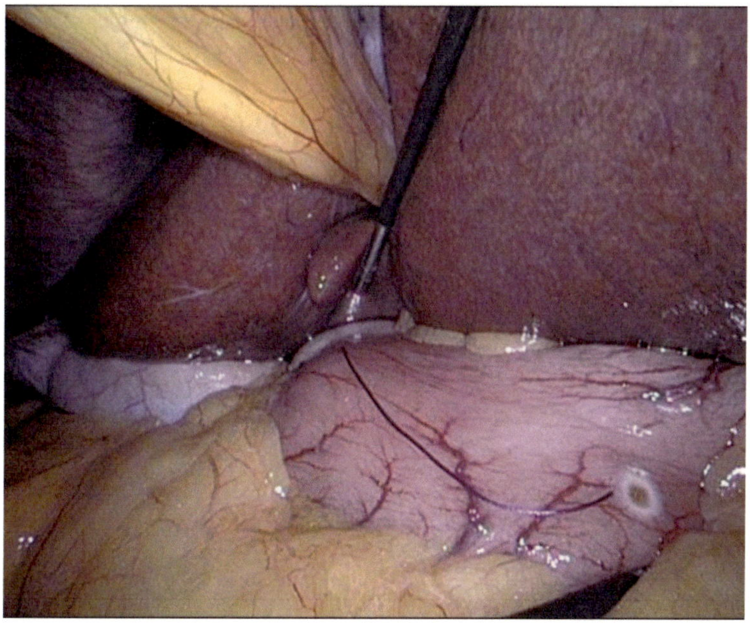

Figure 4. Measuring antral pouch

e. Devascularization:

In the lateral technique, the devascularization process is continued up the greater curve of the stomach to the short gastric vessels with the help of the assistant who maintains traction and exposure during this process (Figure 5a&b). Eventually, one reaches the left crus which is an important landmark of dissection (Figure 6). The left crus muscle is then routinely dissected and hiatus explored by some for a hernia, while others may differ. We selectively explore the hiatus of the symptomatic and endoscopically proven hiatus hernia as all our patients are evaluated for symptoms of reflux by questionnaire pre-operative and also have a gastroscopy performed. In patients with hiatus hernia, the hernia should be reduced and the defect repaired.

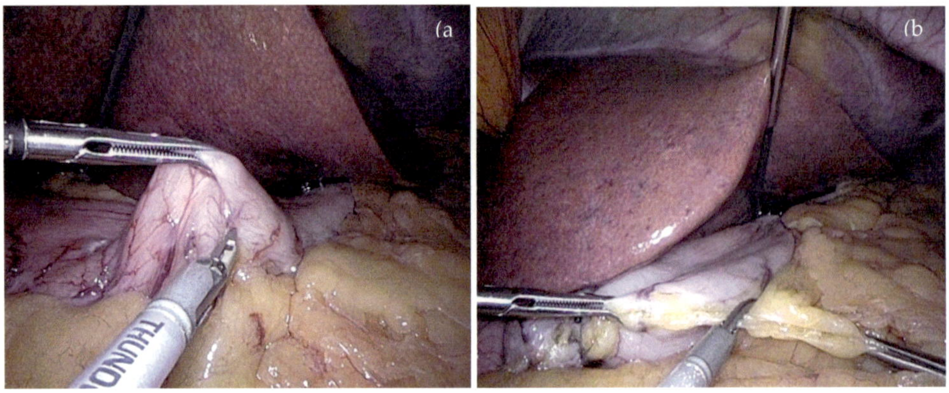

Figure 5. a) Gaining entry into lesser sac, (b) Division of gastro colic ligament

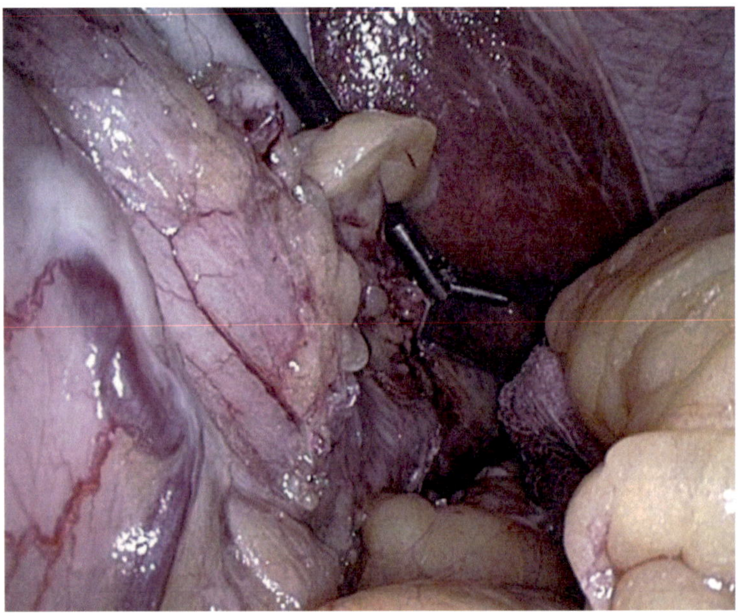

Figure 6. Exposure of left crus of diaphragm

In the medial approach, once the lesser sac is entered the process of stapling starts and devascularization is done only upon completion of sleeve. Dapri et al randomized 20 patients to each arm and looked at the technical outcomes of both medial and lateral approaches; they reported no difference in operative time, preoperative bleeding and hospital stay [16]

f. Gastric tube calibration

The 38 Fr Bougie inserted preoperatively is then advanced into the stomach along the lesser curve. This serves as the border of transection with the linear staple with the remnant lesser curve forming the neo gastric pouch. One of the controversies lies in the optimal size of bougie to be used to size the sleeve. Baltazar uses a 32-French bougie with transection starting at 2-3 cm from the pylorus [17] as opposed to Gagner using a bougie of 60-French bougie and starting the transection at 10 cm away from the pylorus [6]. The bougie size does not affect mean excess weight loss in the short-term but weight loss is significantly different in calibrated sleeves compared to non calibrated sleeve [18]. The meta-analysis of Parikh et al did not show significant difference in %EWL outcomes between bougie <40 Fr and bougie ≥40 Fr up to 36 months (mean: 70.1% EWL; P=0.273) [19]. All panelists in the Expert consensus statement agreed that it was important to use a bougie to size the sleeve and the optimal size of the bougie should be between 32 to 36F [10]. The use of a bougie < 32F may increase postoperative strictures while using bougie of > 36F may bring about limited weight loss effects due to possible dilatation of the sleeve. The size to tube finally achieved will also depend on other factors like over sewing the staple line and whether ones' stapling is snug or lax in relation to the bougie.

g. Creating the gastric tube:

Linear transection of the stomach can be performed using 3.5mm, 3.8 mm or 4.1 mm staples height depending on the thickness of the stomach wall. Any serosal tears during stapling or excessive unexpected bleeding should be carefully evaluated as it may be signaling a poorly stapled area. As the incisura is a common area of narrowing and in indicted for being the cause of the high pressure system resulting in apical leaks in many patients, every effort should be made to stay away and prevent narrowing during stapling. We mark our stapling trajectory with a marker before commencing stapling as over enthusiasm often leads to disasters (Figure 7)

The use of staple-line reinforcement either through suturing or buttressing with biological or synthetic material is a hotly debated topic. Perioperative and postoperative bleeding is a concern for the staple line in sleeve gastrectomy and has been quoted to be between 0 to 14% [20]. Methods to contravene this include the over sewing the staple line with non-absorbable suture material, use of fibrin glue as well as the use of buttressing material along the suture line. Several authors have advocated the use of buttress material to reduce staple line bleeding and leak rates [21], while other reinforcement techniques do not reliably reduce staple line leaks in sleeve gastrectomy [22, 23]. D'Ugo et al. found that in 1162 undergoing LSG, the overall leak rate was 2.8%; Leak rate was lower in patients who had their staple line reinforced with bovine pericardium strips (0.3%) compared to those with synthetic polyester (7.8%) or no reinforcement (4.8%). Postoperative bleeding in patients who had staple line reinforcement was lower (3% vs. 13.7%) [24]

In summary it is suffice to state that current evidence supports the use of buttress material to decrease staple line bleeding [19]. However, buttress material may potentially lower leak rates as it increases burst pressure but the evidence is of poor scientific strength to make a recommendation for their routine use to prevent leaks [23].

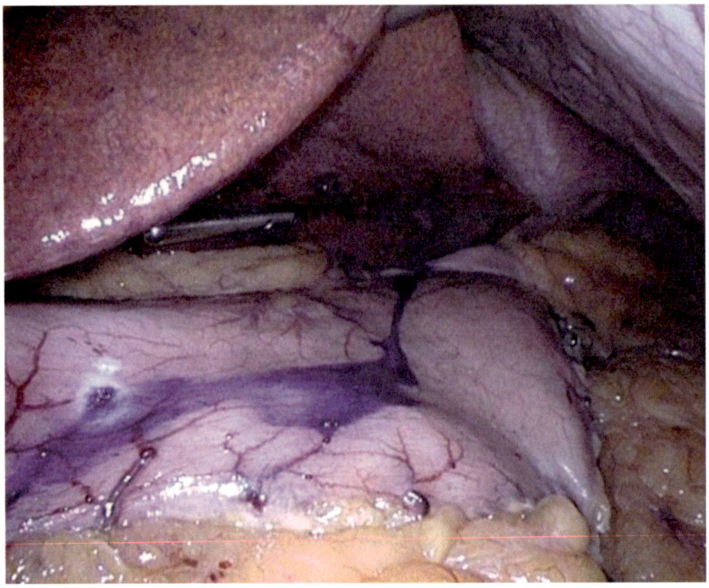

Figure 7. Marking prior to stapling

h. Closure

The specimen is then delivered via the umbilical port (Figure 8). The staple line is then checked for any leaks; we do not routinely oversew the staple line. The 15mm port site is then closed with absorbable suture and the overlying skin stitched with a monofilament absorbable suture after local anesthesia is administered.

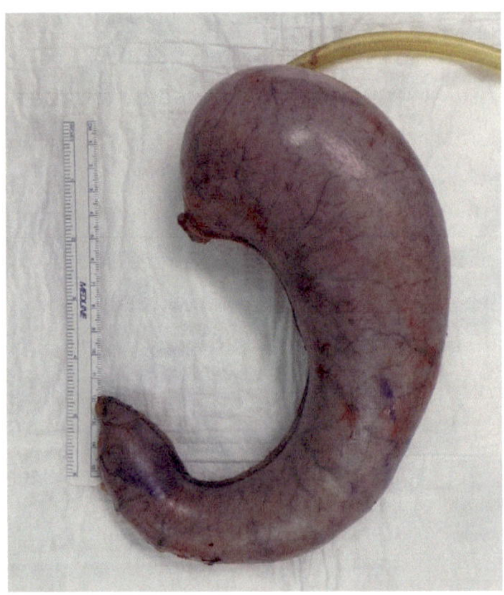

Figure 8. Resected stomach

3. Learning curve

Laparoscopic sleeve gastrectomy looks easy to perform, but yet is a technically demanding procedure; it has to learned through proctorship and mentorship. LSG can be safely and efficiently performed in a newly established bariatric center following a mentorship program. Proficiency seems to require 68 cases. The operative time and hospital stay may significantly decrease with experience early in the learning curve, as opposed to mortality and morbidity rates, conversion rate, and %EWL which will likely remain unchanged [25].

3.1. Post-operative care

For our team, a standardized post operative pathway not only ensures quality care for patients but also help juniors on call staff managing patients strategize management and know who to call when the need arises. We stratify patients based on their ASA grade and the anesthesia team will dictate their admission to intensive care, high dependency or general ward post-operatively. We have standard pain control protocol to prevent narcotic overdose and yet provide effective pain relief.

Clear fluids and ambulation are started on the day of surgery. Patients are reviewed by the dietician and post-operative diet reinforced prior to being discharged home. A phone consult is done 24-48hrs after discharge to reinforce hydration and to ensure patients are recovering well. The clinician nurse, surgical team and dietician review patients 1-2 weeks postoperatively as they slowly progress from clear feeds to soft diet within 4-6 weeks. We believe that the main pillars leading to the success of the sleeve is long term nutritional care. Nutrition relies on a professional medical team providing constant, ongoing patient support throughout all the bariatric process stages working side by side. Patients are regularly reviewed by the dieticians to re-enforce diet recommendations. Long-term, they are prescribed vitamin supplements as advocated by the American Society of Bariatric and Metabolic Surgery guidelines for post bariatric surgery patients [26]. Patients are educated on the need for regular follow up, alike other batriatric procedures. Keren D et al reported improved weight loss and better comorbidity outcomes for those with regular follow up. A total 119 patients were followed up for 30 months with the mean percentage of excess BMI loss being 82.08 ± 9.83 kg for the follow up group and 74.88 ± 8.75 kg for those without follow up [27].

3.2. Complications and management

Chang SH et al reported that the mortality rate for all bariatric procedures within 30 days was 0.08% (95% CI, 0.01%-0.24%); the mortality rate after 30 days was 0.31% (95% CI, 0.01%-0.75%) [28]. Mortality after LSG is exceedingly rare, the 30 days mortality being 0.11% and 1 year mortality of 0.21% [29]. The 30 day morbidity of sleeve gastrectomy is 5.61% which is higher in comparison to the laparoscopic adjustable gastric band of 1.44% but similar to that of the gastric bypass of 5.91% [29].

While the general complications of bariatric procedures remain unchanged among procedures, we will discuss important complications specific to sleeve gastrectomy. Staple line leakage, strictures, and gastrointestinal reflux are the most common complications after LSG.

3.2.1. Leak

Staple line leaks can be divided into acute (< 7 days), early (1-6 weeks), late (after 6 weeks) and chronic (after 12 weeks) [10]. The risk of a leak after LSG was quoted to be 2.4% with 89% of these leaks occurring in the proximal third of the stomach near the angle of His [30]. The pathophysiology of post sleeve is multifactorial and include

a. Tissue Ischemia from

  i. Excessive devascularisation resulting in ischemia of tissue near angle of His

  ii. Removal of fat pad at angle of His

b. Faulty stapling technique

  i. Use of improper staple height leading to poor B formation of staples

  ii. Stapling across esophageal fibers at gastroesophageal junction muscle fibers

c. Functional or anatomical obstruction of gastric tube further increasing intra-gastric pressure of an already elevated pressure system. The sleeve is considered a high pressure tube because there are anatomical sphincters at both ends i.e. the lower esophageal sphincter and the pylorus. This can be contributed by

i. Creation of a gastric tube that is not cylindrical shape as shown in the last three drawing of figure 9 results in a high pressure being built at the proximal most corner of the staple line based on Laplace Law and thus higher chances of leak at the proximal 1/3rd of the tubular stomach

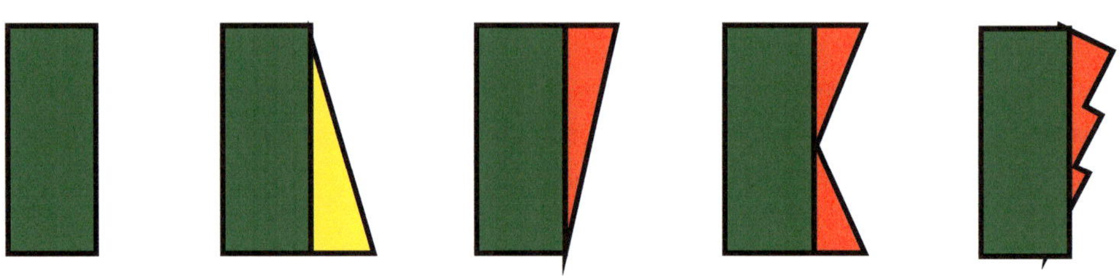

Figure 9. Possible shapes of sleeve created by improper stapling

ii. A staple line that is spiral shaped can result in functional obstruction of the sleeve and a high pressure system develops

iii. Stapling too close to the incisura results in anatomical narrowing, a preventable cause of leak

iv. Post sleeve gastrectomy the tubular sleeve can acquire various shapes-"S" or "L" shape that can potential result in a high pressure system.

A detailed discussion of leak management is beyond the scope of this chapter. The diagnosis of a leak can be made clinically where patients have fever, tachycardia and abdominal pain. The diagnosis can be confirmed with a computerized tomography scan of the abdomen and pelvis or a oral contrast study like gastrograffin meal (Figure 10) The management of the patients with suspected leaks depends first, on whether these patients are haemodynamically stable. In patients who are well with small contained leaks, non-operative management with percutaneous radiological drainage, endoscopic stenting and supportive therapy with antibiotics and total parenteral nutrition has been demonstrated to be effective [31]. In patients who are septic and suspected to have contained or uncontained leaks, immediate operation for washout and drainage of the contaminated field is indicated. These patients will need nutritional support via total parenteral nutrition (TPN), or enteral nutrition via a feeding jejunostomy inserted at time of emergency surgery (preferred option) or naso-jejunal feeding tube. The following interventions (Figure 11) have been described as options in management of simple sleeve leak but they have to be individualized to circumstances and resources at individual centers. For more complex leaks with pleural, bronchial and pulmonary fistulae, detailed discussion with the thoracic surgeon is needed prior to intervention.

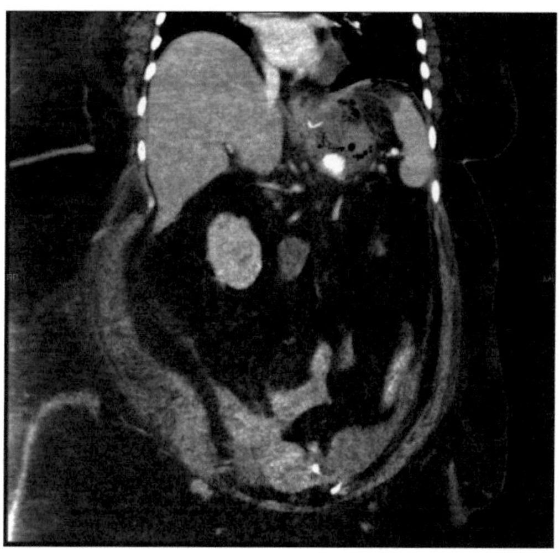

Figure 10. CT scan showing collection and leak of contrast from a proximal sleeve leak

1. Simple suture repair
2. Suture repair with omental patch+/-pyloroplasty
3. El Hassan et al. described a novel method of cannulating a leak site via endoscopy and laparoscopy with a T tube in patients presenting with early leaks, therefore converting the leak site into a controlled fistula together with wide drainage of the abdominal cavity [32].

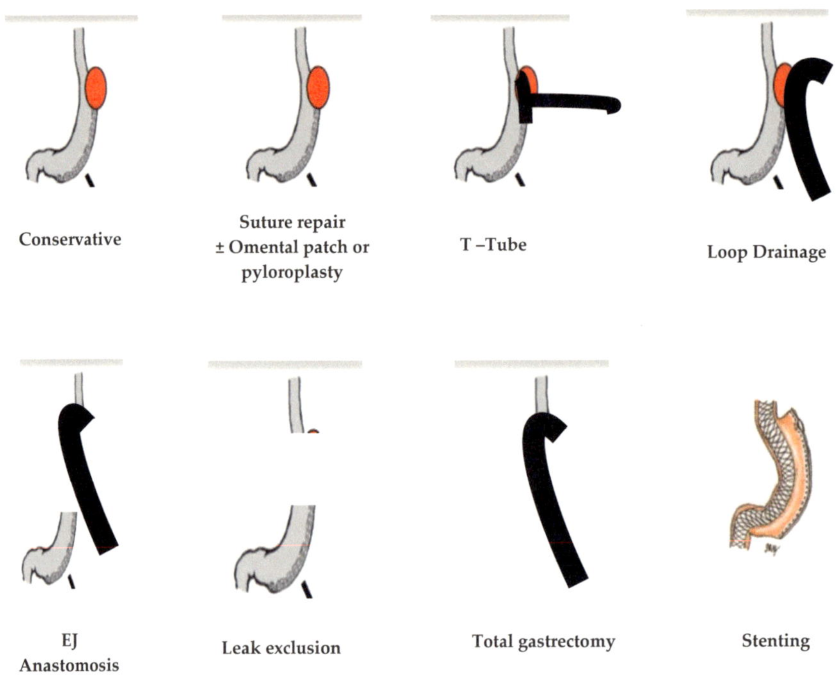

Figure 11. Approaches to sleeve leak

4. Loop drainage: using a free loop of jejunum anastomosed to the leak site

5. Transection of gastroesophageal junction and proximal esophago-jejunostomy leaving gastric tube in place

6. Total gastrectomy with esophago-jejunostomy

7. However currently the most favored approach for acute leak is stenting. Baltazar first reported the use of coated self-expanding stents (CSES) in patients with gastric leaks post sleeve gastrectomy; successful resolution of the leak was reported in 4 out of the 5 patients who underwent CSES. None out of 5 patients required a re-operation and all patients recovered within 6 to 8 weeks. In our opinion early stenting help because stenting

   a. Obliterates the defect thus preventing on going leak and thus helps control sepsis

   b. Neutralises pressure in the stomach as it traverses gastroesophageal junction to across pylorus

   c. It corrects any abnormal axis along the sleeved tube especially acute bends at incisura

   d. Promotes healing by allowing tissue apposition and omental adherence

   e. Reduces the risk of gastro-atmospheric fistula formation

   f. Prevents on going air leak into abdominal cavity in patients who need BIPAP support.

8. For chronic leak with small cavities, endoscopic septoplasty of the bridging stomach wall can be considered

9. Use of tissue glue for closure of chronic fistula

10. Use of endoscopic vacuum therapy (Endosponge) is now a novel approach to upper gastrointestinal tracts and well as the over the scope clips [33].

3.2.2. Strictures / Gastric volvulus

The formation of strictures and gastric pouch stenosis is an uncommon but important complication of LSG. The mean stricture rate in a meta-analysis of 4888 patients who have undergone LSG was 0.5% [30]. Regurgitation is the most common presenting complaint for patients with significant stenosis with the most common site of stenosis at the angular incisura. A smaller bougie size used to size the sleeve is associated with a greater risk for developing of strictures post operatively. In patients whom strictures are suspected, assessment can be via contrast swallow studies or endoscopy. The latter also allows for dilatation to be performed in the same setting. After gastroscopy in patients with short segment stenosis dilatation with or with out stenting is an option, should they respond to this treatment repeat dilatation is advisable. In cases of failed dilatation therapy or long segment stenosis, revisional surgery in the form of conversion to other procedures like gastric bypass or stricturoplasty may be considered. Eubanks reported that in patients who underwent stenting for strictures, 84% achieved immediate symptomatic control and subsequent resolution of the stricture. 16% (1 out of 6 patients) had unsuccessful stent treatment [34, 35]. Burgos also reported success in the use of endoscopic balloon dilatation (preferably a Rigilflex balloon) and endoscopic bougie dilatation in the treatment of stricture post sleeve gastrectomy [34]. In patients with excessive length of stricture where endoscopic dilatation was not possible, Dapri reported that laparoscopic seromyotomy enabled patients to tolerate regular diet with improvement in mean dysphagia score. The aim of the procedure was to achieve a myotomy 1 cm beyond the stenosis proximally and distally [36]. Conversion to a roux-en-Y bypass is the last resort for patients with strictures post sleeve gastrectomy. Other options include stricturoplasty, gastro-gastrostomy and gastrectomy [37].

Gastric volvulus post sleeve gastrectomy is a rare complication. After sleeve gastrectomy the stomach has no fixation along its greater curve, this together with the increased laxity of tissue after weight loss increases the risk of a gastric volvulus. Classically patients present with the Borchardt clinical triad of epigastric pain, retching and inability to pass a nasogastric tube. Laparoscopic fixation of the gastric tube as one would do for congenital malrotation of the stomach will fix the problem.

3.2.3. Gastroesophageal reflux disease (GERD)

In patients with symptoms of pre-existing reflux prior to surgery, Roux-en-Y bypass should be the treatment of choice instead of sleeve gastrectomy. A recent review of the Bariatric Outcomes Longitudinal Database with 4832 patients concluded that LSG did not reliably relieve or improve GERD symptoms and that preoperative GERD was associated with worse outcomes and decreased weight loss with LSG and thus may be a relative contraindication [12]. Institutional practices may vary; some like ours do routine preoperative gastroscopy to establish any reflux esophagitis and exclude the presence of hiatus hernia and if a hiatal hernia is found we would in asymptomatic patients suture repair the hiatal hernia, the surgeon should actively look out for a hiatal hernia intraoperatively and repair the hernia if it is identified. [10] Soricelli et al compared their obese patients with GERD undergoing sleeve with or without hiatal hernia repair and reported 80.4% versus 57.9% remission of GERD and persistent GERD in 7.5% versus 42.2% respectively [38].

The notion that sleeve gastrectomy is a refluxogenic operation remains controversial, as Chiu S et al reviewed 15 published reports of which 4 found sleeve to increase reflux and 7 showed reduction in prevalence of GERD [39]. The anatomic and physiological factors influencing GERD after sleeve gastrectomy are listed as such

a. Worsen GERD

Decrease in gastric emptying

Lower LES pressure

Blunting angle of HIS

Decrease in gastric compliance and volume

Increase gastric pressure

Dilated proximal sleeve (technical) and fundus regeneration,

Angulation, volvulus of sleeve

Gastric atony

b. GERD Improvement

accelerated gastric emptying

weight loss

reduced acid production

removal of fundus (Source of relaxation waves to LES)

Reduced wall tension (Laplace's Law)

In patients who develop reflux symptoms after sleeve gastrectomy, the first line treatment should be with proton pump inhibitors [10]. Early reports have shown that in patients with GERD but refuse gastric bypass, laparoscopic Nissen fundoplication with gastric plication may be an acceptable weight loss option but long-term weight loss data is still required [40].

3.2.4. Nutritional complications

As LSG is a relatively young operation, there is a lack of reliable data arising from long-term follow up of patients who have undergone the procedure. Being a restrictive procedure, it is postulated that no long-term nutritional deficiencies should result from laparoscopic sleeve gastrectomy unless there is inadequate intake of nutrients. If a large sleeve has been resected, Vitamin B12 and resultant megaloblastic anaemia may result due to the lack of Intrinsic factor produced by the remnant stomach. In a cross sectional study reported during a mean follow up period of 4 years post gastric bypass or LSG, patients were identified with several micronutrient deficiencies, including vitamin D, folate, and vitamin B12. LSG had a more favorable effect on the metabolism of vitamin B12 compared with gastric bypass [41]. Thus, postoperative prophylactic iron and B_{12} supplementation, in addition to general multivitamin and mineral supplementation, is recommended based on the comparable deficiency risk.

4. Outcomes

4.1. Weight loss

A meta-analysis in 2012 comprising of 12,129 patients showed that mean percentage of excess weight loss (EWL) at 12 months follow up was 59.0% [42], and this further increased to 64.5% and 66.0% at 24 and 36 months follow up respectively [42]. At 48 months follow up, %EWL declined to 60.9% but this decline was not statistically significant. The same paper also elucidated that patients who underwent Laparoscopic Roux-en-Y bypass had significantly higher %EWL at 12 months follow up but this difference was negligible at 24 months. In a recent review of European data, mean excess weight loss was 68.4%, and 67.4% after 1 and 2 years respectively. Excess weight loss peaked at 70.5% at the 4-year mark before decreasing to 58.3% at the 5-year mark. The authors concluded that the long-term results regarding weight loss were satisfactory [43]. Among super obese patients, the reported mean EWL is be 52%, 43%, 46% at 72, 84 and 96 months follow up respectively [44].

Durability of LSG has been debated and available data does suggest that it is durable. A review of 492 patients with follow-up of at least 5 years after laparoscopic sleeve gastrectomy (373 at 5 years, 72 at 6 years, 13 at 7 years, and 34 at 8 or more years) was performed by Daimantis T at al [45]. Mean preoperative body mass index in all 16 studies was 49.2 kg/m^2. The mean percentage excess weight loss (%EWL) was 62.3%, 53.8%, 43%, and 54.8% at 5, 6, 7, and 8 or more years after LSG, respectively [45]. The overall mean %EWL (defined as the average %EWL at 5 or more years after LSG) was 59.3% (12 studies, n=377 patients). The overall attrition rate was 31.2% (13 studies). They concluded that the existing data supports the role of LSG in the treatment of morbid obesity. It seems to maintain its well-documented weight loss outcome at 5 or more years postoperatively, with the overall mean %EWL at 5 or more years after LSG still remaining in excess of 50%.

4.2. Eating behavior

Several studies had elicited a change of eating behavior following bariatric surgery. Schweiger et al [46] studied the effect of different bariatric operations on food tolerance and quality of eating. On a score of 1 to 27 with 27 points standing for excellent quality of eating, there was no significant difference between patients who underwent RYGB, LAGB, SG and BPD at 3-6 months follow-up. At 6-12 months and long-term follow-up, patients who underwent sleeve gastrectomy achieved a score of 22.27+/-4.66 and 20.25+/-4.9 respectively. Adjusting for other variables, the total score in the 3 follow up periods was 20.1 for RGYB, 14.3 for LAGB, 19.7 for SG and 21.6 for BPD/DS patients. Food tolerance at 2-4 years post surgery was also shown to be best after LSG, followed closely by RYGBP [47].

4.3. Quality of life

In a study of 78 consecutive patients who underwent LSG subjected to the Medical outcomes Study Short Form Questionnaire (SF-36) coupled with the Impact of Weight on Quality of Life-Lite Questionnaire pre-operatively and 12 months post-operatively, scores show a significant overall improvement of the scores 12 months post operatively [48]. Subset analysis showed that lesser patients reported improvement in self-esteem if they suffered complications as a result of the surgery or had negative or moderate loss of weight compared to those who had excellent or satisfactory loss of weight [48]. Studies have also shown that the perceived quality of life after LSG is better compared to LAGB [47, 49]. However, LSG is the only truly irreversible procedure.

5. Sleeve as a metabolic procedure

a. Proposed mechanisms of T2 DM remission

Multiple studies have recently demonstrated that patients with raised BMI and diabetes experience remission of T2DM after laparoscopic sleeve gastrectomy. In a meta-analysis of 27 studies including 673 patients by Gill et al [50], it was shown that DM resolved in 66.2% of patients and improved in another 26.9% with a mean decrease of 1.7 in HbA1c after sleeve gastrectomy at mean follow up of 13 months. Perathoner et al reported a resolution rate of 85% and 50% for Type 2 diabetes mellitus and dyslipidemia respectively in his patients [51]. LSG has been shown to be superior to intensive medical therapy in the resolution of comorbidities and improved quality of life [52].

The mechanism behind T2DM remission following LSG has not been clearly defined. It has been postulated that decreasing oral intake and decreasing insulin resistance instead of increase in insulin secretion is the reason behind T2DM remission. It has been found that in patients who underwent sleeve gastrectomy, their postprandial levels of glucagon like peptide (GLP-1) and total peptide YY (PYY) levels increased significantly at 6 weeks post operation and remained elevated for at least 1 year [53]. By reducing the volume of the stomach, chyme could theoretically be exposed to the L cells earlier in the small bowel earlier, resulting in earlier production of hind gut hormones. Melissas J et al in their gastric emptying study demonstrated faster gastric emptying after sleeve gastrectomy [54]. It has also been postulated that there is restoration of the first phase of insulin secretion after sleeve gastrectomy. N Basso et al reported his "Gastric hypothesis" that a loss in HCL in the stomach stimulated release of GRP which in turn stimulates the release of GLP-1 [55]. GLP-1 initiates what is known as the incretin effect, which increases insulin secretion while inhibiting glucagon release, thereby leading to better glucose hemostasis.

Ghrelin, an appetite stimulant, produces the orexigenic (appetite stimulating) effects via stimulation of neuropeptide Y from the hypothalamus. Ghrelin is mainly produced by the oxyntic cells of the stomach, and has been implicated in obesity and metabolic syndrome. Diet induced weight loss raises circulating ghrelin levels. In sleeve gastrectomy patients, ghrelin levels was markedly reduced and remained low for several months after the operation. The reduction in serum ghrelin levels persisted at five year follow-up post sleeve gastrectomy [56].

Ghrelin not only increases one' appetite but also has counter insulin effects which causes increased insulin resistance. A decrease in ghrelin levels hence, would partly explain improved glucose hemostasis in post SG patients [57]. Most authors would agree that the effect of T2 DM resolution is not due to solely one hormone, but the added effects of appetite suppression and regulation of foregut (e.g. ghrelin) and hindgut (e.g. GLP-1) hormones resulting in improved glucose control overall. PYY a hormone co-secreted with GLP 1 from the distal intestine after meals. It increases insulin sensitivity and also inhibits the hypothalamic production of neuropeptide Y. PYY levels are increased after either sleeve gastrectomy or gastric bypass [58].

b. Metabolic outcomes

Increasingly, more trials have demonstrated the effectiveness of SG for excess weight loss. Himpens et al reported the percentage excess weight loss (EWL) after sleeve gastrectomy as 77.5% and 57.3% at 3 and 6 years respectively [59].

Direct comparison of medical versus bariatric surgical management of obesity and diabetes was performed in the STAMPEDE prospective randomized controlled trial at the Cleveland Clinic [60]. Gastric bypass (Roux-en-Y) or sleeve gastrectomy provided a mean percentage reduction in weight from baseline of 24.5±9.1% and 21.1±8.9% respectively, versus 4.2±8.3% in the intensive medical group. Regarding diabetes, the success rate for reduction in HbA1c to 6.0% at 36 months was met by 5% of the patients in the medical-therapy group, as compared with 38% of those in the gastric-bypass group ($P<0.001$) and 24% of those in the sleeve-gastrectomy group ($P=0.01$) respectively). As a result, lesser medications for diabetes, hypertension and hyperlipidaemia were needed with composite improvement in all parameters of metabolic syndrome. Long-term follow up of sleeve gastrectomy patients at 6-8 years showed a 77% improvement or remission of diabetes [44].

Apart from T2 DM remission, LSG patients also have improved overall cardiovascular risk profiles with improved in dyslipidemia as well as improved blood pressure control.

A systematic analysis of 33 studies comprising 3997 patients demonstrated reduction in hypertension in 75% of cases, with resolution in 58%, at an average follow up of 16.9±9.8 months [61]. Cardiac remodeling following sleeve gastrectomy has been shown on echocardiography. Reduced left ventricular mass, septum and posterior wall thickness, was demonstrated in the study by Cavarretta et al, resulting in improvement in cardiac function [62]. Lipid profile improvement, specifically HDL and triglyceride levels, total cholesterol/HDL and triglyceride/HDL ratios at one year follow-up have been reported without lowering of total cholesterol and LDL levels after sleeve gastrectomy [63].

The Asian population in general is known to develop metabolic syndrome at lower BMIs in comparison to their Caucasian counterparts and hence, studies have reported outcomes from Asia in this cohort. In Asian populations with T2DM and non-morbid obesity (BMI 25-35kg/m^2), sleeve gastrectomy has demonstrated up to 50% resolution in diabetes at 1 year [64]. The principal mechanism is thought to be related to calorie restriction and weight loss, and C-peptide levels returning to >3ng/ml appears to be the most reliable marker of resolution.

5.1. Sleeve gastrectomy as a revisional procedure

Revising a restrictive procedure to yet another revisional procedure and even more to the same procedure does not sound promising to many. However for patients where technical failure has led to failure to lose weight or weight regain, re-sleeve is an option. Rebibo L et all reported 15 patients undergoing repeat sleeve and compared to 30 matched primary sleeve patients. The weight loss for the re-sleeve group was 66% versus 77% for the primary sleeve group at 12 months, which was deemed similar [65]. Cheung et al reviewed the literature on procedures after failed sleeve and concluded that re-sleeve was associated with good weight loss and its technically less challenging nature may make its clinical use more acceptable [66].

Also, sleeve for failed gastric band and vertical banded gastroplasty is a good and effective revisional procedure with 60% EWL at 26 months follow up [67]. Where sleeve took off as a first stage procedure of duodenal switch, it is also finding its way as a first stage procedure for conversion of failed gastric bypass to duodenal switch and has been shown to be safe and effective, leaving patients in better condition to have a duodenal switch [68].

5.2. Sleeve gastrectomy in combination with other bariatric procedures

Gastric bypass has a long history and long-term results support its efficacy in treating obese patients with metabolic disorders. It is an established fact that there are mechanisms beyond weight loss that are responsible for the excellent metabolic outcomes of gastric bypass and that these are related to bypassing the foregut. In order to maximize the scope of sleeve gastrectomy as a metabolic procedure, innovative procedures possessing benefits of both sleeve gastrectomy and gastric bypass are being employed. The sleeve duodeno-jejunal bypass surgery (LSG/DJB), single-anastomosis duodeno-jejunal bypass with sleeve gastrectomy (SADJB-SG), sleeve gastrectomy with loop bipartition, and loop duodeno-jejunal bypass with sleeve gastrectomy, are all largely based on manipulation of foregut. The short-term outcomes have been promising . However, they are still considered experimental as both intermediate and long term data are awaited. Loop duodenal bypass in combination with sleeve gastrectomy for type II diabetes in individuals with BMI 21-38kg/m^2, has shown promising early results, with 91% of achieving HbA1c of 7.0g/dl at 6 months from surgery [69].

Laparoscopic Roux-En-Y gastric bypass prohibits visualization of the excluded stomach. For populations with a high risk of gastric cancer, including Japan, the ability to perform endoscopic visualization after bariatric surgery is paramount. In obese individuals with risk factors such as Helicobacter pylori infection, atrophic gastric mucosa including intestinal metaplasia, or a family history of gastric cancer, Kasama et al. published a series of laparoscopic sleeve gastrectomy with duodeno-jejunal bypass [70]. The procedure was found to be feasible, and safe, with similar EWL to Roux-En-Y gastric bypass. Additional EWL compared to sleeve gastrectomy was attributed to the added malabsorptive effects of the duodenojejunal bypass.

Sleeve with ileal interposition is an example of sleeve with hindgut manipulation. Patients undergoing this procedure have demonstrated restoration of insulin sensitivity, with increased insulin output, and doubling of β-cell glucose sensitivity [71]. The mechanism is postulated to be intestinal over-stimulation, with increased GLP-1 and incretin secretion.

Acknowledgements

A vote of thanks for my dear friend Dr Suthep Udomsawaengsup from Chula Minimally Invasive Surgery Center, Department of Surgery, Faculty of Medicine, Chulalongkorn University,Bangkok,Thailand who has been very instrumental in providing ideas and shared his wisdom with me. My sincere appreciation to my colleague Dr Pradeep Durai for the artwork he has done. I could have not completed this work with out the support of my family and would like to thank them for allowing me to take time off to complete this chapter.

Author details

Asim Shabbir[1,2*] and Jun Liang Teh[1]

*Address all correspondence to: suras@nus.edu.sg

1 Department of Surgery, National University Hospital, Singapore

2 Department of Surgery, National University of Singapore, Singapore

References

[1] Buchwald H, Oien DM. Metabolic/bariatric surgery worldwide 2011. Obes Surg 2013;23:427-36.

[2] Lomanto D, Lee WJ, Goel R, et al. Bariatric surgery in Asia in the last 5 years (2005-2009). Obes Surg 2012;22:502-6.

[3] Hess DS, Hess DW. Biliopancreatic diversion with a duodenal switch. Obes Surg 1998;8:267-82.

[4] de Csepel J, Burpee S, Jossart G, et al. Laparoscopic biliopancreatic diversion with a duodenal switch for morbid obesity: a feasibility study in pigs. J Laparoendosc Adv Surg Tech A 2001;11:79-83.

[5] Ren CJ, Patterson E, Gagner M. Early results of laparoscopic biliopancreatic diversion with duodenal switch: a case series of 40 consecutive patients. Obes Surg 2000;10:514-23; discussion 524.

[6] Gagner M, Rogula T. Laparoscopic reoperative sleeve gastrectomy for poor weight loss after biliopancreatic diversion with duodenal switch. Obes Surg 2003;13:649-54.

[7] Regan JP, Inabnet WB, Gagner M, et al. Early experience with two-stage laparoscopic Roux-en-Y gastric bypass as an alternative in the super-super obese patient. Obes Surg 2003;13:861-4.

[8] Gastrointestinal surgery for severe obesity: National Institutes of Health Consensus Development Conference Statement. Am J Clin Nutr 1992;55:615S-619S.

[9] Malapan K, Goel R, Tai CM, et al. Laparoscopic Roux-en-Y gastric bypass for nonobese type II diabetes mellitus in Asian patients. Surg Obes Relat Dis 2014.

[10] Rosenthal RJ, International Sleeve Gastrectomy Expert P, Diaz AA, et al. International Sleeve Gastrectomy Expert Panel Consensus Statement: best practice guidelines based on experience of >12,000 cases. Surg Obes Relat Dis 2012;8:8-19.

[11] El-Hadi M, Birch DW, Gill RS, et al. The effect of bariatric surgery on gastroesophageal reflux disease. Can J Surg 2014;57:139-44.

[12] DuPree CE, Blair K, Steele SR, et al. Laparoscopic sleeve gastrectomy in patients with preexisting gastroesophageal reflux disease : a national analysis. JAMA Surg 2014;149:328-34.

[13] Ziegler O, Sirveaux MA, Brunaud L, et al. Medical follow up after bariatric surgery: nutritional and drug issues. General recommendations for the prevention and treatment of nutritional deficiencies. Diabetes Metab 2009;35:544-57.

[14] Theodorou D, Doulami G, Larentzakis A, et al. Bougie insertion: A common practice with underestimated dangers. Int J Surg Case Rep 2012;3:74-7.

[15] Michalsky D, Dvorak P, Belacek J, et al. Radical resection of the pyloric antrum and its effect on gastric emptying after sleeve gastrectomy. Obes Surg 2013;23:567-73.

[16] Dapri G, Vaz C, Cadiere GB, et al. A prospective randomized study comparing two different techniques for laparoscopic sleeve gastrectomy. Obes Surg 2007;17:1435-41.

[17] Baltasar A, Serra C, Perez N, et al. Laparoscopic sleeve gastrectomy: a multi-purpose bariatric operation. Obes Surg 2005;15:1124-8.

[18] Weiner RA, Weiner S, Pomhoff I, et al. Laparoscopic sleeve gastrectomy--influence of sleeve size and resected gastric volume. Obes Surg 2007;17:1297-305.

[19] Parikh M, Issa R, McCrillis A, et al. Surgical strategies that may decrease leak after laparoscopic sleeve gastrectomy: a systematic review and meta-analysis of 9991 cases. Ann Surg 2013;257:231-7.

[20] Shi X, Karmali S, Sharma AM, et al. A review of laparoscopic sleeve gastrectomy for morbid obesity. Obes Surg 2010;20:1171-7.

[21] Daskalakis M, Berdan Y, Theodoridou S, et al. Impact of surgeon experience and buttress material on postoperative complications after laparoscopic sleeve gastrectomy. Surg Endosc 2011;25:88-97.

[22] Chen B, Kiriakopoulos A, Tsakayannis D, et al. Reinforcement does not necessarily reduce the rate of staple line leaks after sleeve gastrectomy. A review of the literature and clinical experiences. Obes Surg 2009;19:166-72.

[23] Glaysher M, Khan OA, Mabvuure NT, et al. Staple line reinforcement during laparoscopic sleeve gastrectomy: does it affect clinical outcomes? Int J Surg 2013;11:286-9.

[24] D'Ugo S, Gentileschi P, Benavoli D, et al. Comparative use of different techniques for leak and bleeding prevention during laparoscopic sleeve gastrectomy: A multicenter study. Surg Obes Relat Dis 2014;10:450-4.

[25] Zacharoulis D, Sioka E, Papamargaritis D, et al. Influence of the learning curve on safety and efficiency of laparoscopic sleeve gastrectomy. Obes Surg 2012;22:411-5.

[26] Allied Health Sciences Section Ad Hoc Nutrition C, Aills L, Blankenship J, et al. ASMBS Allied Health Nutritional Guidelines for the Surgical Weight Loss Patient. Surg Obes Relat Dis 2008;4:S73-108.

[27] Keren D, Matter I, Rainis T, et al. Getting the most from the sleeve: the importance of post-operative follow-up. Obes Surg 2011;21:1887-93.

[28] Chang SH, Stoll CR, Song J, et al. The effectiveness and risks of bariatric surgery: an updated systematic review and meta-analysis, 2003-2012. JAMA Surg 2014;149:275-87.

[29] Hutter MM, Schirmer BD, Jones DB, et al. First report from the American College of Surgeons Bariatric Surgery Center Network: laparoscopic sleeve gastrectomy has morbidity and effectiveness positioned between the band and the bypass. Ann Surg 2011;254:410-20; discussion 420-2.

[30] Aurora AR, Khaitan L, Saber AA. Sleeve gastrectomy and the risk of leak: a systematic analysis of 4,888 patients. Surg Endosc 2012;26:1509-15.

[31] Casella G, Soricelli E, Rizzello M, et al. Nonsurgical treatment of staple line leaks after laparoscopic sleeve gastrectomy. Obes Surg 2009;19:821-6.

[32] El Hassan E, Mohamed A, Ibrahim M, et al. Single-stage operative management of laparoscopic sleeve gastrectomy leaks without endoscopic stent placement. Obes Surg 2013;23:722-6.

[33] Rudolf Mennigen NS, Mike G Laukoetter. Novel treatment options for perforations of the upper gastrointestinal tract: Endoscopic vacuum therapy and over-the-scope clips. World Journal of Gastroenterology 2014;20:7767-7776.

[34] Burgos AM, Csendes A, Braghetto I. Gastric stenosis after laparoscopic sleeve gastrectomy in morbidly obese patients. Obes Surg 2013;23:1481-6.

[35] Eubanks S, Edwards CA, Fearing NM, et al. Use of endoscopic stents to treat anastomotic complications after bariatric surgery. J Am Coll Surg 2008;206:935-8; discussion 938-9.

[36] Dapri G, Cadiere GB, Himpens J. Laparoscopic seromyotomy for long stenosis after sleeve gastrectomy with or without duodenal switch. Obes Surg 2009;19:495-9.

[37] Vilallonga R, Himpens J, van de Vrande S. Laparoscopic management of persistent strictures after laparoscopic sleeve gastrectomy. Obes Surg 2013;23:1655-61.

[38] Soricelli E, Iossa A, Casella G, et al. Sleeve gastrectomy and crural repair in obese patients with gastroesophageal reflux disease and/or hiatal hernia. Surg Obes Relat Dis 2013;9:356-61.

[39] Chiu S, Birch DW, Shi X, et al. Effect of sleeve gastrectomy on gastroesophageal reflux disease: a systematic review. Surg Obes Relat Dis 2011;7:510-5.

[40] Lee WJ, Han ML, Ser KH, et al. Laparoscopic Nissen Fundoplication with Gastric Plication as a Potential Treatment of Morbidly Obese Patients with GERD, First Experience and Results. Obes Surg 2014.

[41] Alexandrou A, Armeni E, Kouskouni E, et al. Cross-sectional long-term micronutrient deficiencies after sleeve gastrectomy versus Roux-en-Y gastric bypass: a pilot study. Surg Obes Relat Dis 2014;10:262-8.

[42] Fischer L, Hildebrandt C, Bruckner T, et al. Excessive weight loss after sleeve gastrectomy: a systematic review. Obes Surg 2012;22:721-31.

[43] van Rutte PW, Smulders JF, de Zoete JP, et al. Outcome of sleeve gastrectomy as a primary bariatric procedure. Br J Surg 2014;101:661-8.

[44] Eid GM, Brethauer S, Mattar SG, et al. Laparoscopic sleeve gastrectomy for super obese patients: forty-eight percent excess weight loss after 6 to 8 years with 93% follow-up. Ann Surg 2012;256:262-5.

[45] Diamantis T, Apostolou KG, Alexandrou A, et al. Review of long-term weight loss results after laparoscopic sleeve gastrectomy. Surg Obes Relat Dis 2014;10:177-83.

[46] Schweiger C, Weiss R, Keidar A. Effect of different bariatric operations on food tolerance and quality of eating. Obes Surg 2010;20:1393-9.

[47] Overs SE, Freeman RA, Zarshenas N, et al. Food tolerance and gastrointestinal quality of life following three bariatric procedures: adjustable gastric banding, Roux-en-Y gastric bypass, and sleeve gastrectomy. Obes Surg 2012;22:536-43.

[48] Fezzi M, Kolotkin RL, Nedelcu M, et al. Improvement in quality of life after laparoscopic sleeve gastrectomy. Obes Surg 2011;21:1161-7.

[49] Alley JB, Fenton SJ, Harnisch MC, et al. Quality of life after sleeve gastrectomy and adjustable gastric banding. Surg Obes Relat Dis 2012;8:31-40.

[50] Gill RS, Birch DW, Shi X, et al. Sleeve gastrectomy and type 2 diabetes mellitus: a systematic review. Surg Obes Relat Dis 2010;6:707-13.

[51] Perathoner A, Weissenbacher A, Sucher R, et al. Significant weight loss and rapid resolution of diabetes and dyslipidemia during short-term follow-up after laparoscopic sleeve gastrectomy. Obes Surg 2013;23:1966-72.

[52] Palikhe G, Gupta R, Behera BN, et al. Efficacy of laparoscopic sleeve gastrectomy and intensive medical management in obese patients with type 2 diabetes mellitus. Obes Surg 2014;24:529-35.

[53] Papamargaritis D, le Roux CW, Sioka E, et al. Changes in gut hormone profile and glucose homeostasis after laparoscopic sleeve gastrectomy. Surg Obes Relat Dis 2013;9:192-201.

[54] Melissas J, Koukouraki S, Askoxylakis J, et al. Sleeve gastrectomy: a restrictive procedure? Obes Surg 2007;17:57-62.

[55] Basso N, Capoccia D, Rizzello M, et al. First-phase insulin secretion, insulin sensitivity, ghrelin, GLP-1, and PYY changes 72 h after sleeve gastrectomy in obese diabetic patients: the gastric hypothesis. Surg Endosc 2011;25:3540-50.

[56] Bohdjalian A, Langer FB, Shakeri-Leidenmuhler S, et al. Sleeve gastrectomy as sole and definitive bariatric procedure: 5-year results for weight loss and ghrelin. Obes Surg 2010;20:535-40.

[57] Peterli R, Steinert RE, Woelnerhanssen B, et al. Metabolic and hormonal changes after laparoscopic Roux-en-Y gastric bypass and sleeve gastrectomy: a randomized, prospective trial. Obes Surg 2012;22:740-8.

[58] Karamanakos SN, Vagenas K, Kalfarentzos F, et al. Weight loss, appetite suppression, and changes in fasting and postprandial ghrelin and peptide-YY levels after Roux-en-Y gastric bypass and sleeve gastrectomy: a prospective, double blind study. Ann Surg 2008;247:401-7.

[59] Himpens J, Dobbeleir J, Peeters G. Long-term results of laparoscopic sleeve gastrectomy for obesity. Ann Surg 2010;252:319-24.

[60] Schauer PR, Bhatt DL, Kirwan JP, et al. Bariatric surgery versus intensive medical therapy for diabetes--3-year outcomes. N Engl J Med 2014;370:2002-13.

[61] Sarkhosh K, Birch DW, Shi X, et al. The impact of sleeve gastrectomy on hypertension: a systematic review. Obes Surg 2012;22:832-7.

[62] Cavarretta E, Casella G, Cali B, et al. Cardiac remodeling in obese patients after laparoscopic sleeve gastrectomy. World J Surg 2013;37:565-72.

[63] Zhang F, Strain GW, Lei W, et al. Changes in lipid profiles in morbidly obese patients after laparoscopic sleeve gastrectomy (LSG). Obes Surg 2011;21:305-9.

[64] Lee WJ, Ser KH, Chong K, et al. Laparoscopic sleeve gastrectomy for diabetes treatment in nonmorbidly obese patients: efficacy and change of insulin secretion. Surgery 2010;147:664-9.

[65] Rebibo L, Fuks D, Verhaeghe P, et al. Repeat sleeve gastrectomy compared with primary sleeve gastrectomy: a single-center, matched case study. Obes Surg 2012;22:1909-15.

[66] Cheung D, Switzer NJ, Gill RS, et al. Revisional Bariatric Surgery Following Failed Primary Laparoscopic Sleeve Gastrectomy: A Systematic Review. Obes Surg 2014.

[67] Jacobs M, Gomez E, Romero R, et al. Failed restrictive surgery: is sleeve gastrectomy a good revisional procedure? Obes Surg 2011;21:157-60.

[68] Dapri G, Cadiere GB, Himpens J. Laparoscopic conversion of Roux-en-Y gastric bypass to sleeve gastrectomy as first step of duodenal switch: technique and preliminary outcomes. Obes Surg 2011;21:517-23.

[69] Huang CK, Goel R, Tai CM, et al. Novel metabolic surgery for type II diabetes mellitus: loop duodenojejunal bypass with sleeve gastrectomy. Surg Laparosc Endosc Percutan Tech 2013;23:481-5.

[70] Kasama K, Tagaya N, Kanehira E, et al. Laparoscopic sleeve gastrectomy with duodenojejunal bypass: technique and preliminary results. Obes Surg 2009;19:1341-5.

[71] De Paula AL, Stival AR, Halpern A, et al. Improvement in insulin sensitivity and beta-cell function following ileal interposition with sleeve gastrectomy in type 2 diabetic patients: potential mechanisms. J Gastrointest Surg 2011;15:1344-53.

Chapter 6

Laparoscopic Adjustable Gastric Banded Plication (LAGBP)

Chih-Kun Huang and Jasmeet Singh

Additional information is available at the end of the chapter

http://dx.doi.org/10.5772/58695

1. Introduction

The acceptance of bariatric surgery among morbidly obese patients is highly credited to the introduction of laparoscopy. It has been proven beyond doubt that in morbid obesity, bariatric surgery remains the mainstay management. [1] Although Roux-en-Y gastric bypass has enjoyed the status of being gold standard bariatric surgery for long, it not only involves creation of a severely restrictive gastric pouch, but also excludes a portion of the small bowel. This puts patients at a high risk of developing nutritional deficiencies and some metabolic complications. [2, 3].

Laparoscopic adjustable gastric banding (LAGB) became popular because of its safety profile but its use has decreased over the last decade due to its unfavourable long term outcomes.[4]. Last decade has seen rise in popularity of laparoscopic sleeve gastrectomy (LSG) and has shown promise in medium term results.[5] However, this procedure has the longest staple line among all bariatric procedures which gives rise to the concerns of staple line leak, bleeding and stricture. Furthermore, post-operative decrease in lower esophageal sphincter pressure has been observed.[6] Talebpour and Amoli introduced plication of greater curvature as an alternative to cutting it and recently published their 12 year results with good outcome. [7] However, the possibility of postoperative weight regain owing to plicated gastric tube dilation remains debatable.

In 2009 we introduced a new bariatric procedure to overcome the concerns raised by LSG, LAGB and plication and named it as laparoscopic adjustable gastric banded plication (LAGBP).[8] It involves dual restriction by combining plication with banding. No cutting of stomach is involved. Plication results in initial rapid weight loss and adjustable band ensures long term maintenance of weight loss. Our case-matched comparative study with

INTECH
open science | open minds

© 2014 The Author(s). Licensee InTech. This chapter is distributed under the terms of the Creative Commons Attribution License (http://creativecommons.org/licenses/by/3.0), which permits unrestricted use, distribution, and reproduction in any medium, provided the original work is properly cited.

LSG, LAGBP showed similar results at 2 years in terms weight loss, comorbidity resolution and complications. [9]

2. Case selection

Indications: As for other bariatric procedures, BMI ≧ 40 or BMI ≧35 with co-morbidity is an indication for surgery.[10] This BMI limit may be reduced by 3 for Asian population as per Asia Pacific surgical criteria; BMI ≧ 37 or BMI ≧32 with co-morbidity. [11]

Thorough pre-operative evaluation should be done as for any other bariatric procedure as per protocols of the institution.

Super-obesity (BMI >50 kg/m2) patients may be better served with a mal-absorptive or combined (LRYGB) procedures.

Large hiatus hernia or severe gastro-esophageal reflux is a relative contra-indication.

Patients who cannot follow-up in the clinic for weight loss monitoring and band adjustments must not be offered this procedure.

Patients allergic to silicon must not be offered LAGBP.

3. Surgical technique

All patients should receive prophylaxis against deep vein thrombosis and antibiotics as per the policy of the hospital before starting the procedure.

A bariatric operating table providing at least 45° of reverse Trendelenburg position is preferable.

Room Setup: Patient lies supine on the table with arms extended. Patient must be fastened to the table to prevent slippage during change of posture. Adequate padding must be ensured. Surgeon stands on the right side, camera-man and first assistant on the left side of the patient. Room set-up is depicted in Figure 1.

Port placement: Four or five ports are used (Figure 2). Pneumo-peritoneum is created using Veress needle. Surgeon's left hand port in right upper quadrant (5mm) and right hand at supra-umbilicus (15mm). 5mm assistant port is in left upper quadrant.

Liver retraction: The left lobe of liver could be retracted by Nathanson liver retractor or elevated using T-shaped liver suspension technique.[12] A silicon or rubber drain attached to 2-0 polypropylene suture on long straight needle is used. Two such suspensions usually suffice. The needle is then passed into the inferior surface of the left lobe of the liver so as to exit at the superior surface. The needle is exteriorized by piercing the anterior abdominal wall. The thread is clamped close to the abdominal wall after lifting the left lobe of liver

http://dx.doi.org/10.5772/58695

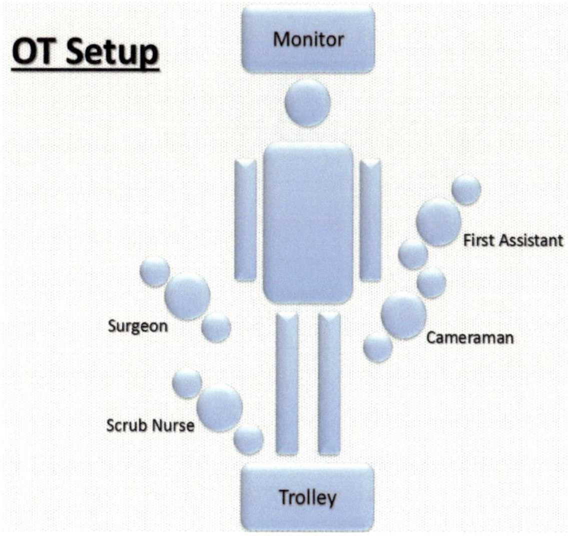

Figure 1. Operation Theater Setup

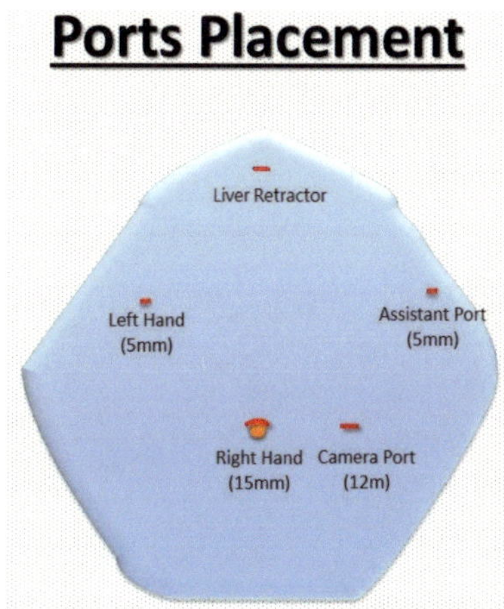

Figure 2. Trocar Placement

Mobilisation of greater curvature: The junction of right and left gastro-epiploic vessels is seen and greater omentum is divided close to the stomach above this point till left crus of diaphragm is clearly seen. Below this point the omentum is divided distal to right gastro-epiploic vessels thereby maintaining venous drainage of the stomach. This helps in decreasing oedema of the stomach wall. Dissection is carried out distally till 3 cm from the pylorus.

Gastric plication formula: Stomach is measured transversely at the level of 6 cm below gastro-esophageal junction (x cm) and plication formula is applied to determine the amount of plication (y=(x+1) / 2). Stomach is marked from lesser curvature side y cm away. (Figure 3)

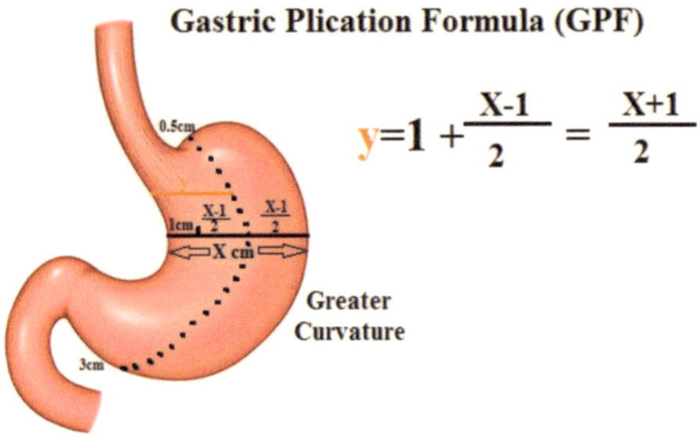

Figure 3. Plication Formula

Plication: It is started from the fundus and progresses towards the pylorus stopping 3 cm from it. The greater curvature is inverted using non-absorbable sutures (2–0 Ethibond Excel Ethicon, St. Stevens-Woluwe, Belgium) at every 2 cm and is then reinforced with a continuous sero-muscular suture (polypropylene 2-0). Second continuous layer is important in preventing the herniation of inverted stomach out of the first layer.

Adjustable band: Band is then inserted using *pars flaccida* technique with minimal dissection and is locked in proper position. The band is checked for proper functioning after its placement. Band need not be fixed to the stomach (Figure 4). The reservoir port is placed over rectus sheath near the umbilicus.

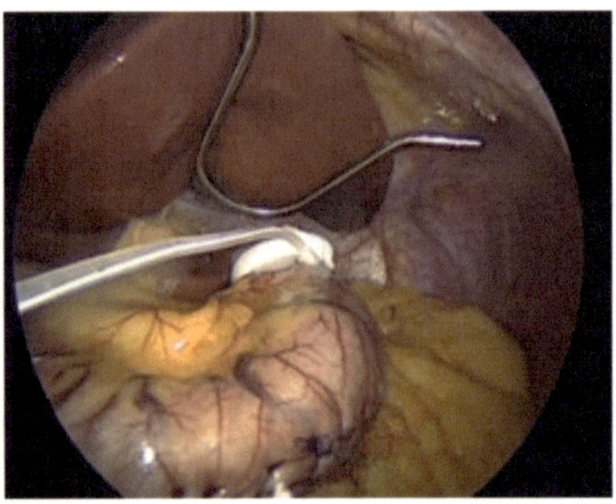

Figure 4. Completed LAGBP

Wound closure: The ports are removed, fascial defects closed and skin is closed with sub-cuticular sutures.

http://dx.doi.org/10.5772/58695

4. Post-operative course

Patients were given oral sips of water 4–6 hours after the surgery. Proton pump inhibitors (PPIs), anti-emetics and dexamethasone are given for 1–2 days.

Patients are discharged if there is no vomiting and they are able to drink enough liquids. Oral PPIs are given for 1 month following surgery.

Liquid diet is prescribed for first week followed by pureed diet for the second week.

This is followed by semi-solid diet for another 2 weeks after which solid food is introduced in a stepwise fashion.

Patient is seen in clinic one week following surgery and thereafter at 1, 3, 6, 9, 12 months. Following which every 6 monthly follow-up is done.

Adjustment of the gastric band is started after 3 months from the surgery if patient complains of less satiety, increased food intake volume or there is inadequate weight loss.

Full evaluation of patient including upper GI endoscopy is performed after 1 year for surveillance and yearly thereafter.

5. Complications

Nausea/vomiting: This can be usually managed with anti-emetics, prokinetics, antacids and adequate hydration.

Acute gastric obstruction: A very tight plication can result in acute gastric obstruction and will require emergent release of plication sutures. This condition settles promptly after the reversal of plication.

Herniation of plicated stomach: May be asymptomatic or may cause acute gastric obstruction presenting with pain, vomiting etc. It may further complicate to ischemia and perforation. Maintaining no more than 2 cm distance between first layer of sutures and a continuous second layer is important to prevent this complication. If symptomatic, surgical correction is necessary by de-plication or re-plication depending upon the condition of the patient.

Perforation peritonitis: This is a rare but serious complication of LAGBP. A high degree of clinical suspicion is important. Pain, tachycardia and high leukocyte count should raise alarm. Computed tomography of abdomen or contrast study may be performed but in the end, clinical judgement must prevail. Laparoscopic exploration should be performed, band removed and plication must be released. Perforation can usually be repaired primarily. However, wedge resection or sleeve gastrectomy may be required for ischemic part.

Band infection: As with LAGB, band may get infected and usually needs removal.

Band adjustment schedule: First adjustment is not done before 3 months from surgery so as to let the oedema subside. Later, patient is followed at intervals as mentioned before and band is adjusted according to weight loss and feeling of satiety.

6. Technical tips

Proper case selection is important. Patients must understand the need for follow-up and band adjustment.

By preserving the right gastroepiploic vessels, the oedema of stomach can be decreased thereby decreasing the post-operative vomiting. And adopting the gastric plication formula could facilitate and standardize the surgery to prevent the complications from over-plication.

Advantages of LAGBP: It avoids cutting of stomach thereby decreasing chances of leak, haemorrhage and stricture. The placement of adjustable band over plication helps in preventing dilatation of stomach over long time. Plication decreases number of band adjustments required for adequate weight loss and hence decreases complications of banding. Stomach wall near cardia is not cut as in LSG and hence may decrease gastro-esophageal reflux. No part of stomach is removed and hence vitamin / mineral deficiencies may be less as compared to LSG.

Proper follow-up is of paramount importance for adequate weight loss.

7. Conclusion

Laparoscopic adjustable gastric banded placation (LAGBP) owns dual effect of plication and band adjustment without side effects of gastrointestinal anastomosis and mal-absorption, proved to be a safe and effective bariatric surgery.

Author details

Chih-Kun Huang and Jasmeet Singh

Bariatric & Metabolic International (B.M.I) Surgery Center, E-Da Hospital, Taiwan

References

[1] Karlsson J, Taft C, Ryden A, et al. Ten-year trends in health-related quality of life after surgical and conventional treatment for severe obesity: the SOS intervention study. Int J Obes. 2007;31:1248–61.

[2] Segaran E. Provision of nutritional support to those experiencing complications following bariatric surgery. ProcNutrSoc 2010;10: 1–7.

[3] D Kumpf VJ, Slocum K, Binkley J, Jensen G. Complications after bariatric surgery: survey evaluation impact on the practice of specialized nutritional support. NutrClinPract 2007;22:673– 8.

[4] Suter M, Calmes JM, Paroz A, Giusti V. A 10-year experience with laparoscopic gastric banding for morbid obesity: high long-term complication and failure rates. ObesSurg 2006;16:829 –35.

[5] Updated position statement on sleeve gastrectomy as a bariatric procedure. soard. 2012.02.001.

[6] Braghetto I, Lanzarini E, Korn O, Valladares H, Molina JC, Henriquez A. Manometric changes of the lower esophageal sphincter after sleeve gastrectomy in obese patients. ObesSurg 2010;20:357– 62.

[7] Mohammad Talebpour, Seyed Mohammad KalantarMotamedi, AtiehTalebpour and HamedVahidi. Twelve year experience of laparoscopic gastric plication in morbid obesity: development of the technique and patient outcomes. Annals of Surgical Innovation and Research 2012, 6:7.

[8] Huang CK, Lo CH, Shabbir A, Tai CM (2012) Novel bariatric technology: laparoscopic adjustable gastric banded plication: technique and preliminary results. SurgObesRelat Dis 8(1):41–5.

[9] Huang CK, Chhabra N, Goel R, Hung CM, Chang PC, Chen YS (2013) Laparoscopic adjustable gastric banded plication: a case-matched comparative study with laparoscopic sleeve gastrectomy. ObesSurg 23(8):1319-23.

[10] NIH conference. Gastrointestinal surgery for severe obesity. Consensus Development Conference Panel. Ann Intern Med. 1991 Dec 15;115(12):956-61.

[11] Lee WJ, Wang W. Bariatric surgery: Asia-Pacific perspective. Obes Surg. 2005;15(6): 751–7.

[12] Zachariah SK, Tai CM, Chang PC, Se AO, Huang CK. The "T-suspension tape" for liver and gallbladder retraction in bariatric surgery: feasibility, technique, and initial experience. J LaparoendoscAdvSurg Tech A. 2013 Apr;23(4):311-5.

[13] Laparoscopic Adjustable Gastric Banded Plication (LAGBP)

Chapter 7

Novel Metabolic/Bariatric Surgery — Loop Duodenojejunal Bypass with Sleeve Gastrectomy (LDJB-SG)

Chih-Kun Huang, Jasmeet Singh Ahluwalia,
Amit Garg, Voraboot Taweerutchana , Andrea Ooi,
Po-Chih Chang and Ming-Che Hsin

Additional information is available at the end of the chapter

http://dx.doi.org/10.5772/58890

1. Introduction

Metabolic surgery is now a well-established concept which originated from diabetic remission of bariatric surgery. Roux-en-Y gastric bypass (RYGB), biliopancreatic diversion with duodenal switch (BPD-DS), mini-gastric bypass (MGB) and even the new entrant, sleeve gastrectomy (SG), have been shown to achieve good results in diabetic control and glycaemia result of type II Diabetes Mellitus. [1, 2, 3, 4] But all these procedures come with their own set of limitations and long-term complications. Marginal ulcer, intractable dumping syndrome, internal herniation, bile reflux, malnutrition are to name a few and some patients require reoperation in the future because of these complications.

Laparoscopic RYGB (LRYGB) has been taken as the gold standard procedure now in the world in treating morbid obese patients with type II Diabetes Mellitus. LRYGB can be accomplished using either an antecolic or retrocolic approach which creates 3 or 2 potential mesenteric defects respectively. Otherwise, internal hernia has been the most common causes of small bowel obstruction following LRYGB, with an incidence ranging from 1% to 9%. [5, 6, 7] It has become ever more frequent following laparoscopic RYGB than it was during open surgery era. [8]

Marginal ulceration has been also reported in 1%–16% of patients. [9] Stricture of the gastrojejunal anastomosis happens in 2.9% to 23.0% of patients. [10, 11] Gastrogastric fistula has been reported in 1.5% and 6.0% of cases. [12]

INTECH
open science | open minds

© 2014 The Author(s). Licensee InTech. This chapter is distributed under the terms of the Creative Commons Attribution License (http://creativecommons.org/licenses/by/3.0), which permits unrestricted use, distribution, and eproduction in any medium, provided the original work is properly cited.

Another rare but potentially devastating complication of RYGB involves the inadvertent anastomosis of the proximal biliopancreatic limb of the jejunum to the gastric pouch in conjunction with a misplaced jejunojejunostomy. [13]

Compared with gastric bypass, duodenal switch could not get rid of all these complications mentioned above and even is associated with a greater risk of vitamin deficiencies. [14] Kevin et al reported that 18% of patients were hypoalbuminemic, 32% anemic, 25% hypocalcemic, and almost half had low vitamin A, D, and K levels, despite more than 80% taking vitamin supplementation. [15]

Though LSG is a simpler procedure and owns satisfactory weight loss, a recent meta-analysis and some randomized controlled trials have demonstrated inferiority of LSG over LRYGB in the treatment of diabetes and control of metabolic syndrome. [16, 17, 18, 19] Evidence suggests that MGB has real risk of bile reflux due to the loop configuration that may have long-term damaging effects to the gastric pouch and possibly cancer of the distalesophagus. [20, 21, 22] McCarthy et al performed endoscopy in 28 patients who had undergone loop gastroenterostomy, loop gastroenterostomy plus diverting enteroenterostomy between the afferent and efferent loops or Roux-en-Y anastomosis. [23] Total bile acid levels in the gastric pouch were 2080. 1 μg/mL in patients who had undergone loop gastroenterostomy alone compared with 165.0 μg/mL in patients who had undergone Roux-en-Y anastomosis. Gastritis by endoscopy was only 13% in Roux-en-Y group compared to 71% in loop gastroenterostomy group. In 2007 Johnson WH et al concluded that MGB does require revision in some patients (because of leak, bile reflux, intractable marginal ulcer, mal-absorption/malnutrition, weight gain etc.) and that conversion to RYGB is a common form of revision. [24]

The never-ending search of a more physiological and less complex surgery has led surgeons to develop novel procedures. "Laparoscopic Loop Duodenojejunal Bypass with Sleeve Gastrectomy (LDJB-SG)" [25] was first invented and described by Chih-Kun Huang since October 2011, which was reported in 2013. The pyloric preserving mechanism could decrease the incidence of dumping syndrome. Also, the mixture of alkaline bile and pancreatic enzyme with gastric acid around anastomosis also decrease the incidence of marginal ulcer. The acid and intrinsic factor secretion would be maintained. Thus, iron, vitamin and protein deficiency should be less because some part of antrumis preserved. Moreover, one anastomosis and only Petersen's defect may help in decreasing the chances of anastomotic leakage and internal hernia as compared to RYGB and BPD-DS. It also eliminates the chances of gastro-gastric fistula with sometimes complicates LRYGB. And less bypassed bowel (200-300 cm) would improve the malnutrition part as compared to BPD-DS.

2. Mechanism of action

LDJB-SG works by combining restriction of food (Sleeve Gastrectomy) with bypassing duodenum and proximal jejunum. This procedure predominantly owned the part of duodenojejunal bypass for glycemic control based on the foregut hypothesis. And sleeve gastrectomy is incorporated into this to eliminate the ghrelin effect to make sufficient weight loss and reversal of insulin resistance. The rapid gastric emptying ensures swifter nutrient delivery to the hindgut with secretion of incretins like GLP-1 which are responsible for augmenting satiety and improving pancreatic function.

Restriction: It is achieved by performing sleeve gastrectomy along a 38 Fr orogastric tube.

Bypass: 200-300 cm of duodenum and proximal jejunum is bypassed.

Special features:

- Single loop duodenojejunal anastomosis other than Roux-en-Y anastomosis could prevent more possibility of anastomotic stricture or leakage.
- Only Peterson defect to decrease the chances of internal hernia.
- Pyloric preservation to avoid dumping syndrome.
- Mixture of alkaline bile and pancreatic enzyme with gastric acid around anastomosis to decrease the incidence of marginal ulcer.
- Less chances of hypo-proteinemia, vitamins deficiency and diarrhoea as compared to BPD-DS which has only 75-100 cm of common limb.
- Easy post-operative endoscopic surveillance of remnant stomach.

2.1. Indications of the procedure

- Body mass index (BMI) ≧ 35 with co-morbidities or BMI ≧ 40
- BMI ≧ 27. 5with poorly controlled Type 2 Diabetes Mellitus (HbA1c >7)

2.2. Contraindications of this procedure

- Chronic alcoholism
- Drug/substance abuse
- Psychiatric disorder
- Severe gastro-esophageal reflux disease
- Chronic duodenal ulcer

2.3. The procedure

a. Preoperative Considerations

The preoperative examination does not differ from other bariatric procedures. The patients are admitted one day before surgery to maintain stable glucose level less than 200mg/dL by insulin infusion if necessary, and keep patients on clear liquid diet one day before surgery. One dose antibiotics (cephalosporin) and 40 mg pantoprazole is given half an hour before surgery. Antithrombotic devise and low molecular weight heparin are prescribed to avoid deep vein thrombosis and thrombo-embolic events.

b. Technique:

- *Positioning:* Patient is laid supine on the table (Figure 1). Surgeon stands on the right side of the patient. Cameraman and first assistant stand on the left of the patient.

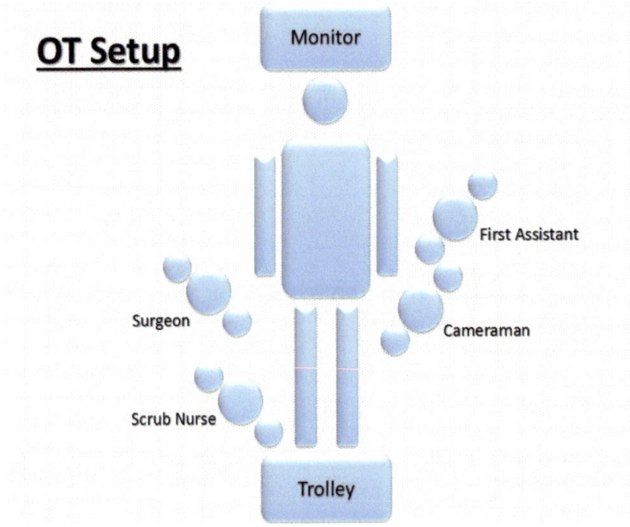

Figure 1. OT Setup

- *Port-positions:* 5 ports technique to access the abdominal cavity as shown in figure 2.

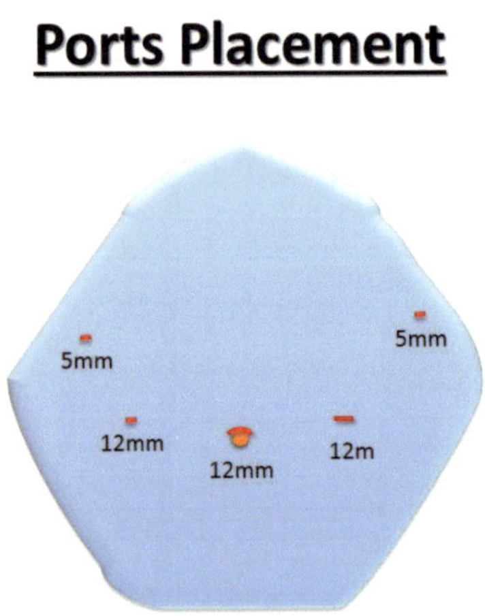

Figure 2. Port Placement

- *Liver retraction:* The liver could be retracted by Nathanson liver retractor or T-shape liver suspension tapes in order to achieve good exposure of both stomach and duodenal area.

http://dx.doi.org/10.5772/58890

- *Sleeve Gastrectomy:* The first step involves devascularisation of greater curvature of stomach, 4 cm from the pylorus till the left crus of diaphragm, using an energy source like LigaSure vessel sealing (Covidien, USA), sealing the gastric branches of gastroepiploic vessels and short gastric vessels. Sleeve gastrectomyis then performed using 38 Fr orogastric tube as a stent with sequential firing of Endo GIA™ 60 mm articulating medium/thick Reload with Tri-Staple™ (Covidien, USA) (Figure 3). Black reloads are used for the first two firings while purple reloads are used for the subsequent firings toward the gastric fundus.

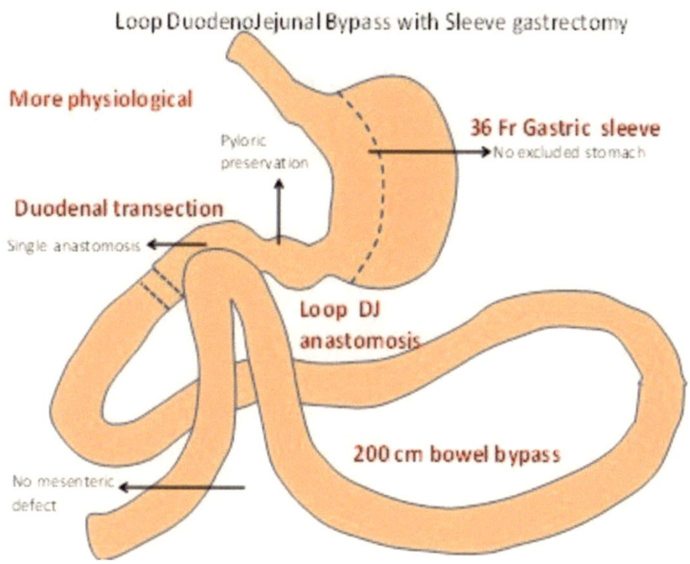

Figure 3. Loop Duodenojejunal Bypass with sleeve gastrectomy

- *Duodenal transaction:* After ensuring haemostasis, a stay suture is placed at the distal end of stomach tube for counter-traction and better visualization of the first part of the duodenum. A tunnel is created posterior to the first part of duodenum 2 cm distal to pylorus using Goldfinger (Ethicon Endo Surgery USA). A tape is passed and lifted cranially and laterally for traction so as to aid in insertion of the stapler. The first part of the duodenumis transected2cm distal to the pylorus with Endo GIA™ 45 mm Curved Tip Articulating Vascular/Medium Reload with Tri-Staple™ (Covidien, USA) and take care not to injure common bile duct, pancreas and major vessels in the area. Routine over-sewing of the distal duodenal stump is not necessary.

- *Duodeno-jejunostomy:* Jejunum is measured for 200-300 cm from the ligament of Treitz. A 1. 5 cm enterotomy is created in jejunum and the first part of duodenum. Iso-peristaltic totally hand-sewn side to side anastomosis is then performed using 3/0 absorbable suture. The air leak test is performed to check the anastomosis. After the anastomosis, we place an antitorsion suture between the antrum and upper jejunum, 4 cm proximal to the duodenojejunostomy.

- *Mesenteric defect closure and drainage:* Peterson's defect is repaired with a continuous non-absorbable suture. Jackson-Pratt drain is placed behind the duodeno-jejunal anastomosis reaching up to the sleeve to complete the procedure.

2.4. Post-operative care

A postoperative antibiotic (Cephalosporin) is given for one day. Deep-breathing exercises, early mobilization and adequate pain control administration are given in order to avoid postoperative pulmonary complications. A clear-liquid diet is started once the patient is fully conscious. The patients are discharged once they can tolerate oral fluid well, which is usually by postoperative day 2-3. Pantoprazole 40 mg is given for 30 days daily after discharge. Patients are scheduled for follow-up in the outpatient clinic 1 week after the discharge. They are advanced to take soft diet by the third week and solid diet intake after 1 month. Subsequent routine follow-ups are done at 1, 3, 6, 9 and 12 months after surgery. Thereafter, patients are advised to visit hospital every 6 months.

3. Complications

Bleeding: This usually happens from the long staple line of sleeve gastrectomy or divided mesentery, but mostly could be managed conservatively. Re-laparoscopy is indicated if the patient presents as persistent drop in hematocrit despite blood transfusion or shock.

Leak: Leakage of sleeve gastrectomy mostly occurs near the upper end of staple line which could be treated initially by stent placement endoscopically and drainage of abscess. And if leakage occurs in anastomosis of duodeno-jejunosotomy, conversion to Roux-en-Y gastric bypass with removal of distal stomach and first part of duodenum would be a rescue procedure.

Stricture: Stricture of sleeve gastrectomy could be managed by endoscopic stent or balloon dilatation, laparoscopic stricturoplasty or conversion to Roux-en-Y gastric bypass.

Internal Hernia: Even we routinely repair Peterson defect during the procedure, but internal hernia is still a possibility to happen. Suspicion should be made when patient presented as intermittent cramping upper abdominal pain or acute/chronic intestinal obstruction. Abdominal CT Scan is mandatory in diagnosis and laparoscopic exploration would be necessary when definite diagnosis is obscure.

4. Micronutrient supplementation after this procedure

We recommended taking two multivitamin tablets each containing B1, B12, folate, iron and vitamin D in a dose of 1.1 mg, 2.4 microgram, 400 microgram, 10-15 mg and 10 microgram respectively and 2000 mg of calcium citrate in two divided doses.

http://dx.doi.org/10.5772/58890

4.1. Surgical results

To compare the safety and diabetic remission and metabolic results after LDJB-SG and RYGB in patients with BMI < 35 kg/m2, we did a prospective non-randomized study starting from July 2006 to March 2012 in Bariatric & Metabolic International Surgery Centre, E-Da Hospital, Taiwan (Table 1). A total of 109 patients were involved with a follow-up period of at least one year. 89 patients underwent Laparoscopic RYGB and 20 underwent Laparoscopic LDJB-SG. Mean age (50.0 ± 8.6 years in LDJB-SG group vs. 50.0 ± 10.6 in RYGB group), BMI (27.9 ± 3.0 vs. 28.9 ± 3.8 kg/m2), FPG (126.0 ± 37.8 vs. 168.0 ± 68.9 mg/dl), HbA1c (7.5 ± 1.8 vs. 9.0 ± 1.9), c-peptide (2.1 ± 1.0 vs. 2.2 ± 1.6ng/ml), and duration of diabetes (78.0 ± 65.5 vs. 84.0 ± 70.1 months) were similar in two groups. Fasting plasma glucose (FPG=126.0 ± 37.8 vs 168.0 ± 68.9 mg/dl) and HbA1c (7.5 ± 1.8 vs. 9.0 ± 1.9 %) were significantly higher in LRYGB group though. Operative time (119.0 ± 46.9 vs. 73.0 ± 51.3 minutes) and length of stay in the hospital (3.0 ± 1.3 vs. 2.0 ± 2.4 days) were significantly higher in LDJB-SG group.

Parameters	**LDJB-SG group**	**LRYGB group**	***P value***
Gender (M/F)	13/7	54/35	0.719
Age (y)	50.0 ± 8.6	50.0 ± 10.6	0.745
BMI (kg/m2)	27.9 ± 3.0	28.9 ± 3.8	0.121
FPG (mg/dl)	126.0 ± 37.8	168.0 ± 68.9	0.002
HbA1c (%)	7.5 ± 1.8	9.0 ± 1.9	0.004
C-peptide (ng/ml)	2.1 ± 1.0	2.2 ± 1.6	0.270
TG (mg/dl)	158.0 ± 182.1	166.0 ± 115.6	0.585
CHO (mg/dl)	182.5 ± 35.6	202.0 ± 193.0	0.039
HDL (mg/dl)	46.0 ± 12.8	45.0 ± 9.8	0.993
LDL (mg/dl)	106.5 ± 245.2	110.0 ± 35.7	0.267
AST (U/L)	35.0 ± 15.5	30.0 ± 38.5	0.666
ALT (U/L)	33.0 ± 29.5	34.0 ± 64.8	0.663
Family history DM (N;%)	12;60%	65;73%	0.247
Duration of DM (month)	78.0 ± 65.5	84.0 ± 70.1	0.064
Operation time (min)	119.0 ± 46.9	73.0 ± 51.3	0.000
LOS (day)	3.0 ± 1.3	2.0 ± 2.4	0.000

BMI: Body Mass Index; FPG: Fasting Plasma Glucose; CHO: Cholesterol; TG: Triglyceride; LOS: Length of Stay

Table 1. Comparison of clinical and biochemical characteristics at baseline between the patients underwent LDJB-SG and RYGB

At one year after surgery, there was no significant difference in BMI (22.5 ± 2.4 in LDJB-SG vs. 21.0 ± 2.7 LRYGB group), HbA1c (6.0 ± 0.9 vs. 6.3 ± 1.2) or c-peptide (1.4 ± 0.5 vs. 1.3 ± 1.5 ng/ml) but FPG was significantly lower (98.0 ± 18.0 vs. 106.0 ± 31.7 mg/dl) in LDJB-SG group (Table 2). There were 17 late complications seen in LRYGB group vs nil in LDJB-SG group during first one year after surgery (Table 3). LDJB-SG had higher remission rate (60% vs. 40%) of diabetes and also better glycemic control (90% vs. 71%) as compared to RYGB (Figure 4).

Parameters	LDJB-SG group	RYGB group	*P value*
BMI (kg/m2)	22.5 ± 2.4	21.0 ± 2.7	0.234
FPG (mg/dl)	98.0 ± 18.0	106.0 ± 31.7	0.048
HbA1c (%)	6.0 ± 0.9	6.3 ± 1.2	0.442
C-peptide (ng/ml)	1.4 ± 0.5	1.3 ± 1.5	0.881
TG (mg/dl)	119.0 ± 81.4	84.0 ± 46.3	0.257
CHO (mg/dl)	180.5 ± 33.7	173.0 ± 39.4	0.339
HDL (mg/dl)	49.5 ± 12.2	52.0 ± 13.7	0.540
LDL (mg/dl)	99.0 ± 20.3	85.0 ± 27.8	0.503
AST (U/L)	24.0 ± 12.1	30.0 ± 38.5	0.157
ALT (U/L)	26.5 ± 21.6	34.0 ± 64.8	0.062

BMI: Body Mass Index; FPG: Fasting Plasma Glucose; CHO: Cholesterol; TG:Triglyceride

Table 2. Comparison of clinical and biochemical characteristics at 1 year between the patients underwent LDJB-SG and RYGB.

	LDJB-SG group (20)	RYGB group (89)
Resolution of co morbidities (%)		
T2DM	60	49
Hypertension	85.7	88.2
Dyslipidemia	70	76.6
Operative complications (N)		
Major	1	1
Late	0	17
Mortality	0	1

T2DM: Type II Diabetes Mellitus

Table 3. Operative outcomes of LDJB-SG and RYGB.

http://dx.doi.org/10.5772/58890

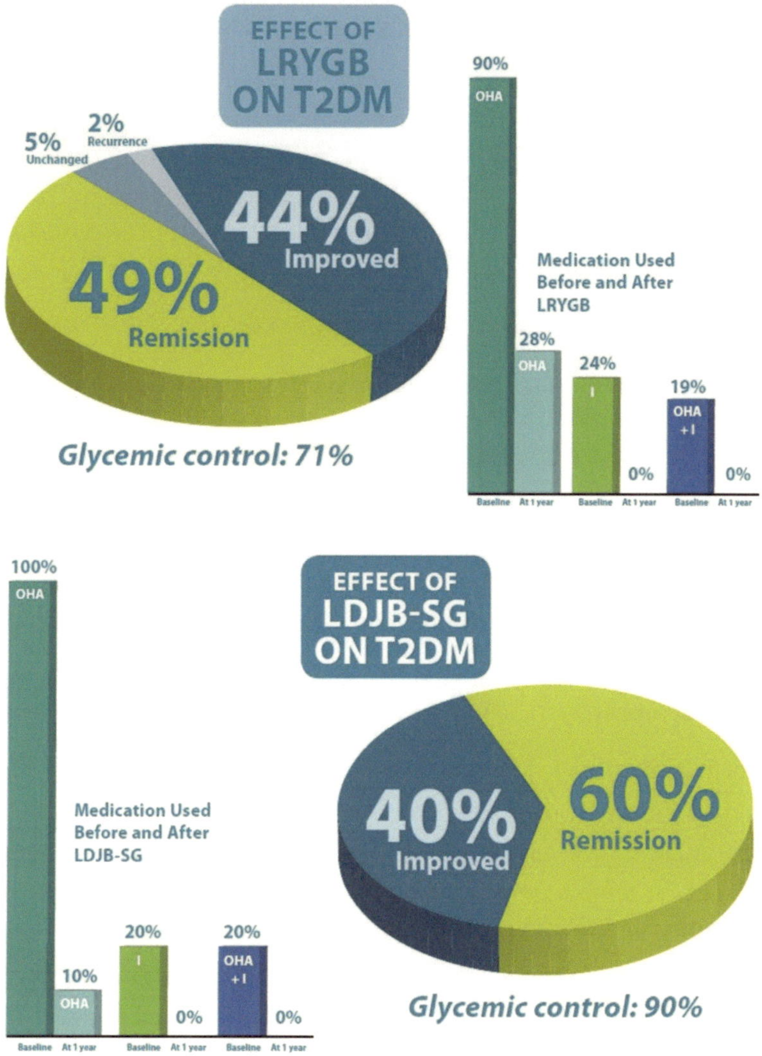

Figure 4. Effect of LRYGB on T2DM

This study concluded that LDJB-SG has higher remission rate and better glycemic control as compared to RYGB in patient with BMI < 35kg/m2.

5. Conclusion

LDJB-SG is a novel metabolic surgery, with single anastomosis and mesenteric defect aimed at achieving less mal-absorption, decreased gastrointestinal complications, adequate weight loss and good remission of T2DM. From the preliminary results of weight loss and glycemic controls, this novel procedure will not only become an important surgical procedure of treating type II D.M in the near future, but also in treating morbid obesity.

Author details

Chih-Kun Huang*, Jasmeet Singh Ahluwalia, Amit Garg, Voraboot Taweerutchana , Andrea Ooi, Po-Chih Chang and Ming-Che Hsin

*Address all correspondence to: dr. ckhuang@hotmail. com

Bariatric & Metabolic International Surgery Centre, E-Da hospital, Taiwan

References

[1] Cohen RV, Pinheiro JC, Schiavon CA, et al. Effects of gastric bypass surgery in patients with type 2 diabetes and only mild obesity. Diabetes Care. 2012;35 (7) :1420–8.

[2] Huang CK, ShabbirA, Lo CH, et al. Laparoscopic Roux-en-Y gastric bypass for the treatment of type II

[3] Scopinaro N, Papadia F, Marinari G, et al. Long-term control of type 2 diabetes mellitus and the other

[4] Eid GM, Brethauer S, Mattar SG, et al. Laparoscopic sleeve gastrectomy for super obese patients: forty-eight percent excess weight loss after 6 to 8 years with 93% follow-up. Ann Surg 2012;256:262-5.

[5] Schnieder C, Cobb W, Scott J, et al. Rapid excess weight loss following laparoscopic gastric bypass leads to increased risk of internal hernia. SurgEndosc. 2011;25:1594–8.

[6] Steele KE, Prokopowicz GP, Magnuson T, et al. Laparoscopic antecolic Roux-en-Y gastric bypass with closure of internal defects leads to fewer internal hernias than the retrocolic approach. SurgEndosc. 2008;22:2056–61.

[7] Paroz A, Calmes JM, Giusti V, et al. Internal hernia after laparoscopic Roux-en-Y gastric bypass for morbid obesity: a continuous challenge in bariatric surgery. Obes Surg. 2006;16:1482–7.

[8] Higa KD, Ho T, Boone KB. Internal hernias after laparoscopic Roux-en-Y gastric bypass: incidence, treatment and prevention. Obes Surg. 2003;13:350–4.

[9] Csendes A, Burgos AM, Altuve J, et al. Incidence of marginal ulcer 1 month and 1 to 2 years after gastric bypass: a prospective consecutive endoscopic evaluation of 442 patients with morbid obesity. Obes Surg. 2009;19:135–8.

[10] Mathew A, Veliuona MA, DePalma FJ, et al. Gastrojejunal stricture after gastric bypass and efficacy of endoscopic intervention. Dig Dis Sci. 2009;54:1971–8.

[11] Alasfar F, Sabnis AA, Liu RC, et al. Stricture rate after laparoscopic Roux-en-Y gastric bypass with a 21-mm circular Stapler: The Cleve-land Clinic Experience. Med Princ-Pract. 2009;18:364–7.

[12] Tucker ON, Szomstein S, Rosenthal RJ. Surgical management of gastro–gastric fistula after divided laparoscopic Roux-en-Y gastric bypass for morbid obesity. J Gastroint-est Surg. 2007;11:1673–9.

[13] Sherman V, Dan AG, Lord JM, et al. Complications of gastric bypass: avoiding the Roux-en-O configuration. Obes Surg. 2009;19:1190–4.

[14] Aasheim ET, Björkman S, Søvik TT, et al. Vitamin status after bariatric surgery: a randomized study of gastric bypass and duodenal switch. Am J ClinNutr 2009;90:15–22.

[15] Dolan K, Hatzifotis M, Newbury L, Lowe N, Fielding G. A clinical and nutritional comparison of biliopancreatic diversion with and without duodenal switch. Ann Surg 2004;240:51– 6.

[16] Jian-Fang Li, Dan-Dan Lai, Bin Ni, Kuan-Xue Sun. Comparison of laparoscopic Roux-en-Y gastric bypass with laparoscopic sleeve gastrectomy for morbid obesity or type 2 diabetes mellitus: a meta-analysis of randomized controlled trials. Can J Surg. Dec 2013; 56 (6) : E158–E164.

[17] Lee WJ, Lee YC, Chen JC, et al. Gastric bypass vs sleeve gastrectomy for type 2 diabetes mellitus: a randomized controlled trial. Arch Surg. 2011;146:143–8.

[18] Kehagias I, Karamanakos SN, Argentou M, et al. Randomized clinical trial of laparoscopic Roux-en-Y gastric bypass versus laparoscopic sleeve gastrectomy for the management of patients with BMI < 50 kg/m2. Obes Surg. 2011;21:1650–6.

[19] Ramón JM, Salvans S, Crous X, et al. Effect of Roux-en-Y gastric bypass vs sleeve gastrectomy on glucose and gut hormones: a prospective randomised trial. J Gastroint-est Surg. 2012;16:1116–22.

[20] Brendan J. Collins, Tomoharu Miyashita, Michael Schweitzer, Thomas Magnuson, John W. Harmon. Gastric Bypass, Why Roux-en-Y? A Review of Experimental Data. ARCH SURG/VOL 142 (NO. 10), OCT 2007.

[21] Kazumori H, Ishihara S, Rumi MAK, et al. Bile acids directly augment caudal related homeobox gene Cdx2 expression in oesophageal keratinocytes in Barrett's epithelium. Gut. 2006;55 (1) :16-25.

[22] Jaiswal K, Lopez-Guzman C, Souza RF, et al. Bile salt exposure increases proliferation through p38 and ERK MAPK pathways in a non-neoplastic Barrett's cell line. Am J PhysiolGastrointest Liver Physiol. 2006;290 (2) :G335-G342.

[23] McCarthy HB, Rucker RD, Chan EK, et al. Gastritis after gastric bypass surgery. Surgery. 1985;98 (1) :68-71.

[24] Johnson WH, Fernanadez AZ, Farrell TM, Macdonald KG, Grant JP, McMahon RL, Pryor AD, Wolfe LG, DeMaria EJ. Surgical revision of loop ("mini") gastric bypass procedure: multicenter review of complications and conversions to Roux-en-Y gastric bypass. SurgObesRelat Dis. 2007 Jan-Feb;3 (1) :37-41.

[25] Huang CK, Goel R, Tai CM, et al. Novel metabolic surgery for Type2 Diabetes Mellitus: Loop Duodenojejunal Bypass with Sleeve Gastrectomy. SurgLaparoscEndoscPercutsn Tech 2013. Dec;23 (6) :481-5.

[26] Novel Metabolic Surgery: Loop duodenojejunostomy with sleeve gastrectomy. (LDJB-SG)